Aus der Klinik für Neurochirurgie

der Universität zu Köln

Direktor: Univ.-Prof. Dr. med. Norfrid Klug

Central Auditory Implants

(Zentrale Hörprothetik)

Habilitationsschrift zur Erlangung der venia legendi

für das Fach Allgemeine Neurochirurgie

an der Hohen Medizinischen Fakultät

der Universität zu Köln

vorgelegt von

Dr. med. Johannes Kuchta

aus Bonn

Köln 2007

1.   Introduction

1.1.   Central auditory implants

For centuries it was a dream of physicians and engineers to implant machines into humans to compensate for a variety of disabilities of the nervous system. Even Galvani or Benjamin Franklin conducted experiments with the application of electrical stimulation to paralyzed muscles. In the last years the field of functional neurorehabilitation with neural prosthesis is evolving fast due to the progress in microelectronics. Already a number of bionic devices are restoring the connections between sound, vision, and the nerve system. The most common prosthesis of this kind is the cardiac pacemaker, although it doesn´t actually stimulate nerve cells but muscle cells. Another electric stimulator has been developed for the phrenic nerve. The phrenic nerve stimulator may help patients with upper spinal cord injury to breathe. Other research concerning motor prostheses enabling paralyzed patients to use their hands or to walk is in progress, but the long-term benefit for the patients is not clear. The most sensitive and problematic part of the systems seems to be not the electronics, but the establishment of a clear and stable electro-neural interface. By far the most successful neuroprosthetic device is the "bionic ear" i.e. the cochlear implant and the auditory brainstem implant (Eisenberg 1987, McDermott 1992, Kuchta 2002).

Prosthetic electrical stimulation of the auditory system has been far more successful than had originally been predicted. With modern implant devices, most deaf people with cochlear implants can understand speech well enough to converse over the telephone. In the past 25 years, prosthetic electrical stimulation has been applied to the cochlear nucleus of patients with no remaining auditory nerve (Brackmann et al, 1993). Although the speech recognition performance of these patients is not as good as in patients with multichannel cochlear implants, the auditory brainstem implant (ABI) provides clear benefit to deaf patients (Shannon et al., 1992, 1993; Otto et al, 1998). Here clinical and laboratory studies in collaboration with the House Ear Institute, Los Angeles will be reported. Research concerning the inferior colliculus as a possible target for prosthetic stimulation was performed together with Chris Schreiner, University of San Francisco and Dough McCreery (the Huntington Memorial Institute, Pasadena). The phrase "central" in "Central auditory implants" refers to targets of implantation proximal to the cochlea. These include primarily the cochlear nucleus and the inferior colliculus.

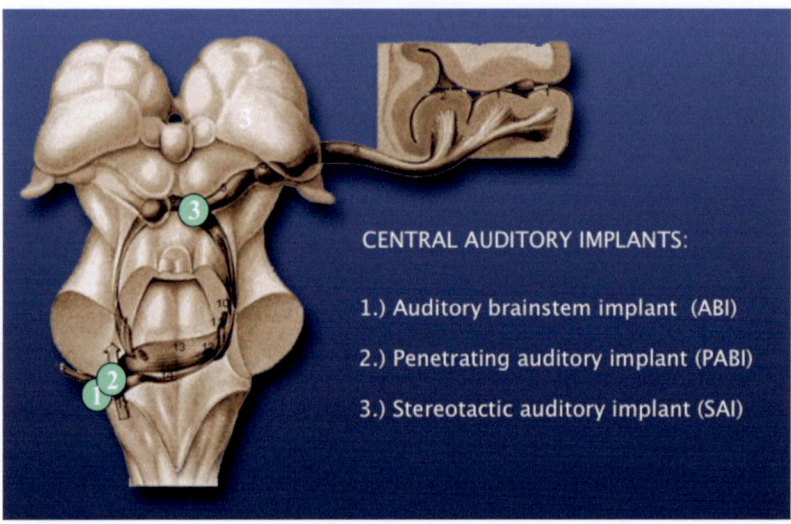

Figure 1: Device and target region for central auditory implantation: 1) The auditory brainstem surface implant (ABI), target point: surface of the cochlear nucleus. 2) Penetrating auditory brainstem implant (PABI), target point: inside ventral cochlear nucleus. 3) Stereotactic auditory implant (SAI), target point: the inferior colliculus. (adapted from interBRAIN, Springer, Heidelberg, Germany, 1998).

1.2.   Mechanisms of speech perception

Speech perception is dependent on both temporal and spectral (frequency) cues. In normal hearing the different frequencies of incoming sounds create a displacement at different points along the basilar membrane of the cochlea. This way the cochlea acts like a spectrum analyzer. It decomposes complex sounds into their frequency components. In auditory implants, the speech processor and the individual electrodes have to take over this task. There has been an intensive discussion in recent years regarding how many individual channels of spectral information are necessary to achieve good consonant and vowel recognition. Though a limited degree of word and sentence recognition is possible even in the absence of spectral cues, a significant intra-individual improvement of perceptual performance has been demonstrated from single-channel to multi-channel electrodes in cochlear implant recipients.

From cochlear implant studies it is known that spectral information is of greater importance for implant listeners in vowel recognition than in consonant recognition (Fu et al., 1999; Shannon et al 1995). There are relatively fewer differences in duration and amplitude among vowels than among consonants. Consonant recognition by implant users may be more dependent on temporal cues than vowel recognition and therefore consonants may be identifiable with less spectral information, i.e. fewer electrodes. The main task in the development of auditory prostheses is to determine which global cues in the sensory peripheral response patterns are most important for cueing the central pattern recognition process and how to convey those cues most effectively.

Historically, speech recognition research has focused on the role of spectral patterns, e.g. formants and formant transitions, in distinguishing phonemes. Physiological studies have also focused on frequency based speech cues. Recent speech recognition results in cochlear implant patients (Fishman et al., 1997), and acoustic experiments with reduced spectral cues (Shannon et al., 1995) have shown that high levels of speech recognition are possible with only minimal spectral cues. Only three broad spectral bands (or electrodes) are necessary for 90% correct recognition of words in sentences in cochlear implants.

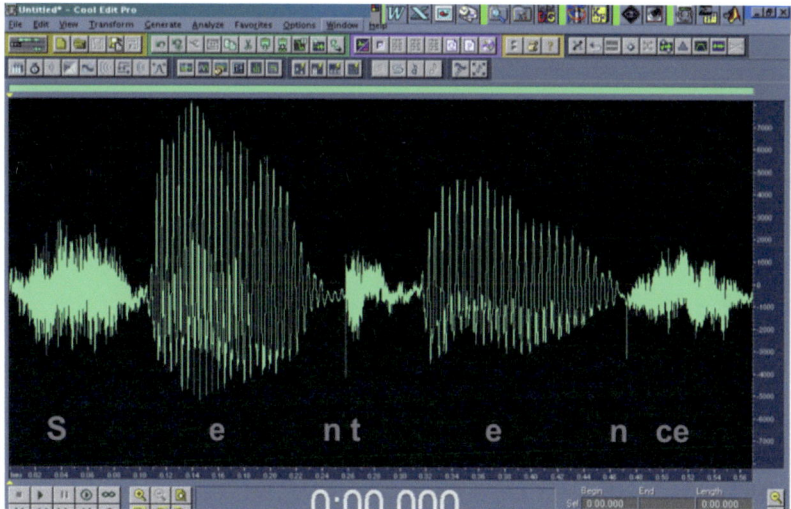

Figure 2: "Screenshot" from a recording of the word "sentence" ("Cool edit" audio software). Vowels ("e") and different consonants ("s, t, n, c") can be visually recognized by their wave form characteristics. Here only the amplitude of the different sounds composing the word "sentence" is displayed. Due to the high plasticity and pattern recognition capabilities of the brain some degree of speech recognition is possible on the basis of temporal pattern recognition alone.

How much spectral information is necessary to understand speech? Must spectral information be presented to the correct tonotopic region of neurons to be useful? Is the brain flexible enough to utilize the patterns of speech information even if it is coupled to the tonotopic dimension of the auditory nervous system in a nonlinear manner? These questions are as yet unanswered and the answers are critical for the optimal design of auditory prostheses. These questions are even more important for the application of central auditory implants than in cochlear implants. In chapters 3.1.1.- 3.1.4., answers for these questions will be provided on the basis of postoperative ABI test results.

In a patient who has a complete survival of auditory nerves and their peripheral processes (dendrites) and in which the array of electrodes is well positioned relatively to the nerve, each electrode would activate a distinct group of neurons and each electrode would yield a distinct and unique pitch percept. The envelope information from several frequency bands is used to modulate pulses that are applied to the electrodes. In this case each sector of neurons receives a portion of the envelope information from speech. The sectors are properly ordered, so that the envelopes from lower frequency spectral regions are presented to more apical neurons. However, even in this case the neurons are not excited by the envelope information that is appropriate for their "characteristic frequency". Thus, envelope information from low frequency regions of speech is presented to neurons that would normally respond to considerably higher frequencies. Nevertheless, most cochlear implant patients understand speech quite well. In a patient with poor nerve survival and/or poor placement of the electrode array, most of the electrodes may activate the same population of neurons. The patient may perceive little if any pitch difference across the array of electrodes. The pitch elicited by an electrode in any location can be high or low, depending on the "characteristic frequency" of the remaining nerve fibers. In this case, the patient would probably have limited capacity to recognize speech, and the actual nerve fibers stimulated would depend on the location of the surviving nerves, the position of the electrodes, and the current flow pathway. This patient would not recognize speech well, but it is not clear which factor (non-homogeneous tonotopic mapping, broad overlap/interaction between electrodes, etc.) would contribute most heavily to the poor performance. Speech processor adjustments (e.g., re-ordering electrodes in pitch order to compensate for a non-tonotopic electrode pitch) may improve speech recognition to some degree in such a case. The cochlear nucleus contains many anatomically and functionally distinct subunits. Each subunit has its own tonotopic organization, and little is known about the importance of the intrinsic processing in each subunit. In addition, the orientation of the tonotopic axis of each subunit is different from the others. In January 2001 it was not clear which subunit would be the preferred target region for a penetrating microelectrode. Some answers to this question will be provided in chapter 3.2.1 (concluding that the ideal target for prosthetic neurostimulation is the ventral cochlear nucleus). An additional concern for penetrating microelectrodes, even if they can activate the tonotopic organization in a selective manner, is that direct electrical stimulation of the cochlear nucleus might bypass some intrinsic neural processing that is essential for speech.

Even in the best case, penetrating microelectrodes may not activate evenly spaced tonotopic regions. In an individual patient, for example, most electrodes might stimulate a relatively low-pitch region, while only a few might stimulate higher-pitch regions. Speech processors would probably need to accommodate this non-uniform electrode spacing to optimize speech performance, all of which makes the postoperative "hook-up" and programming in ABI patients much more problematic than in Cochlear implant patients.

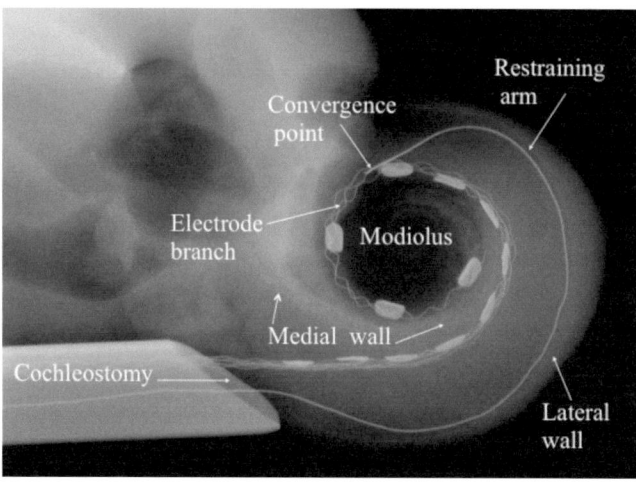

Figure 3: X-ray of a cochlear implant in a laboratory setting. The tonotopic organisation of the cochlear is reflected in the programming of the different electrodes implanted with high frequencies represented at the basal turn and deep frequencies represented at the distal end (apical turn) of the cochlea (Neuroanatomic Lab, House Ear Institute, Los Angeles, USA).

1.3.   Functional aspects in auditory rehabilitation

In cochlear implants, the electrodes are located in the scala tympani in the basal turn of the cochlea. Electrodes are generally aligned along the tonotopic axis of the nerves. Most researchers assume that successful speech recognition is possible only if the electrodes excite distinct nerve populations that produce distinctive pitches.

Initially, auditory researchers assumed that artificial (electrical) stimulation of the auditory system would not be very useful because the pattern of neural activity would be highly unnatural. Electrical stimulation cannot recreate the complex temporal and spatial patterns of neural activity that exist in a normal ear. However, cochlear implants, while producing an unnatural and artificial pattern of nerve activity, do allow for considerable speech recognition. We now know that the reason for this apparent discrepancy is the powerful pattern recognition capability of the human brain. A sensory prosthesis does not have to reproduce all of the details of the peripheral activity pattern to be useful. While we understand details of the peripheral pattern quite well, and while those details may play a role in fine auditory discriminations, they are clearly not all necessary for recognition of speech. Because listeners must be able to understand speech in a broad range of acoustic conditions and by a wide range of speakers and speaking styles, speech pattern perception is largely a higher order cognitive function not critically dependent on all details of the peripheral pattern of nerve activity.

The first auditory brainstem implantation was performed in 1997 by Dr. Bill Hitselberger at the House Ear Institute (HEI) in Los Angeles, California, USA in a patient with neurofibromatosis type 2 (NF2, see chapter 2.2). After removal of the vestibular schwannoma the electrode (a simple bipolar ball electrode) was inserted into the cochlear nucleus and connected transcutaneous to an external cable. A microphone and an external processor was attached. Postoperatively the patient was able to perceive auditory information when stimulated. Interestingly, this first implant can also be considered as the first penetrating deep brain auditory implant. All patients that were following received multipolar plate electrodes that did not penetrate the brainstem parenchyma, but were implanted on the surface of the brainstem in contact to the cochlear nucleus. Until November 2005, more than three hundred patients with NF2 have received an auditory brainstem implant (ABI) worldwide. About half of these patients (125) were operated between 1979-2005 at HEI, where the original device was developed by Drs. William House and William Hitselberger. In most of these patients the ABI is able to provide auditory sensations useful in recognizing environmental sounds and improving communication significantly in conjunction with lipreading. Present technology produces electrical stimulation of the human cochlear nucleus through surface electrodes placed in the lateral recess of the IV ventricle (chapter 2.4) adjacent to the ventral and dorsal cochlear nucleus: VCN/DCN (Brackmann et al, 1993; Shannon et al., 1993; Otto et al., 1998).

1.4.   Auditory rehabilitation in Neurofibromatosis Type 2

Neurofibromatosis Type II is a genetic condition that affects one in 40,000 people in the United States. Individuals develop benign tumors on both auditory nerves and may have to have both hearing nerves severed by tumor removal. When this occurs, profound deafness may result as hearing aids or cochlear implants will be of no assistance. HEI developed the FDA-approved multichannel auditory brainstem implant (ABI) device to provide useful sound information to these individuals. NF2 patients may also develop multiple tumors on the other cranial nerves (associated with swallowing, speech, eye movements, facial sensation) and on the spinal nerves. In 1987, the National Institute of Health Consensus Development Conference on NF developed the guidelines for the diagnosis of NF2 as distinct from Neurofibromatosis Type 1. NF2 is characterized by bilateral acoustic neuromas (or vestibular schwannomas (VS)) with multiple meningiomas, cranial tumors, optic gliomas, and spinal tumors (Gutmann et al., 1997). A definitive diagnosis is made on the basis of the presence of bilateral vestibular schwannomas, or unilateral vestibular schwannoma by the age of 30 and a first-degree relative with NF2, or at least two of the following conditions known to be associated with NF2: meningioma, glioma, schwannoma, or juvenile poster subcapsular lenticular opacity/juvenile cortical cataract (Gutmann et al., 1997). There is much heterogenity in the presentation of the disease and in the genetic mutation linked to the manifestations of the disease. Within a family, the expression of NF2 tends to be very much the same (Parry et al., 1994). This indicates a large genetic component to the disease with much variability within parameters in the observed phenotype. Studies (Evans et.al., 1998, Kluwe et al., 1996; Ruttledge et al, 1996) have shown that a truncating mutation ("nonsense mutation") is linked with the more severe form of NF2. The more severe form ("Wishart") is very disabling due to unrelenting growth of schwannomas and meningiomas from childhood, resulting in blindness, deafness, paralysis, and often death by the age of 40.

Despite the strong genotype-phenotype correlation, individual differences in tumor growth occurs within subjects, making it difficult to predict how an individual tumor will change over time even when the genotype is known. The mild, or "Gardner," form of NF2 is less debilitating. The schwannomas may remain the same size for years, only few meningiomas will develop. The patient may not become symptomatic until late in life, and will have fewer disabilities (Baser et. al., 1996; Bijlsma et. al., 1995; Evans et. al., 1998; Gardner et. al., 1930; Kluwe et. al., 1996; Mautner et. al., 1996; Parry et. al., 1994; Sainio et. al., 1995; Welling, 1998; Wishart, 1822). Bilateral acoustic neuromas (histologically and more exactly: vestibular schwannomas) are benign neoplasms of the acoustic or 8th cranial nerve (Cushing, 1917). The tumors typically are located on the superior vestibular nerve at the glial-Schwann cell junction (Obersteiner- Redlich zone) within the internal acoustic meatus. Symptoms of vestibular schwannoma growth may include: dizziness, imbalance, tinnitus, hearing loss progressing to deafness, facial nerve paralysis, brainstem compression and death. Patients tend to be diagnosed with NF2 around age 25 after experiencing symptoms of the disease for an average of 7 years. Before the invention of the ABI, all NF2 patients became completely deaf either due to their progressive bilateral tumor growth, or as a result of translabyrinthine surgery for the removal of the tumor. Cochlear implants or other more conventional hearing aids are not an option in these patients because the deafening lesion is proximal (central) to the cochlear and the middle ear structures thereby causing a disconnection of the 8th nerve before entering the brain.

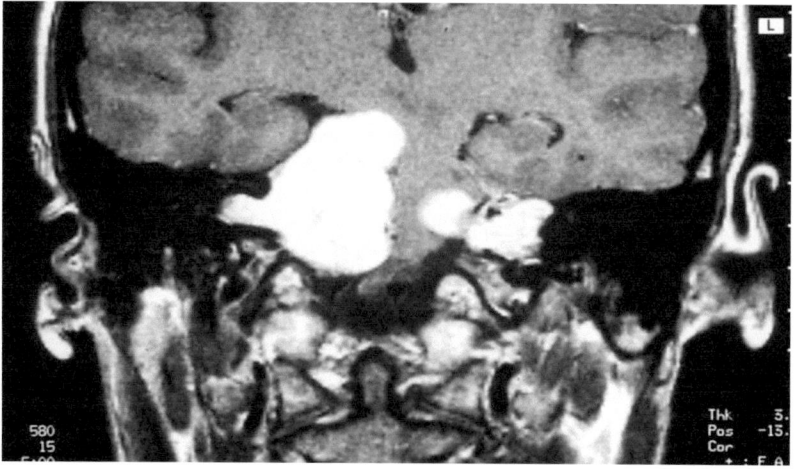

Figure 4: T1-weightened MRI Image (coronar section) in a NF2 patient showing significant bilateral brainstem compression due to huge vestibular schwannomas.

1.4.1. Technical details of the ABI surface device

The ABI works in the following manner (Figure 5): Sounds are picked up by a small microphone located close to the external ear. A thin cord carries the sounds from the microphone to a miniaturized speech processor. The speech processor filters and analyzes the sounds, and digitizes it into coded signals. The coded signals are sent through a thin cable from the speech processor to the transmitting coil. The transmitting coil sends the coded signals as radio signals to the implant under the skin. The implant (receiver/stimulator device, R/S, Figure 6) delivers the appropriate electrical signals to the set of electrodes (electrode array) on the cochlear nucleus in the brainstem. The electrodes stimulate the cochlear nucleus, producing responses that can be interpreted by the brain as sound. The multichannel ABI is MRI compatible up to 1.5 Tesla, as long as the magnet is removed from the R/S. This allows recipients of the NUCLEUS-device to receive follow up MR imaging.

With the Med-El Combi 40+ABI device implanted, MRI scans can be performed safe and feasible in a 1.5 T MRI (Behr and Hofmann, 2006). Behr and Hofmann were able to obtain good-quality diagnostic images of the head and the spine in 5 implanted NF-2 patients with the Med-El device. In conventional T1-weighted spin echo sequences the posterior fossa of the operated side was distorted with a large susceptibility artefact. The parameters of the implant remained unchanged after the MRI examiniation and no negative effect on patients could be observed. The ABI system includes the capability to stimulate between any pair of electrodes on the array (bipolar mode), or the use of a remote electrode as ground (monopolar mode/ chapter 2.6).

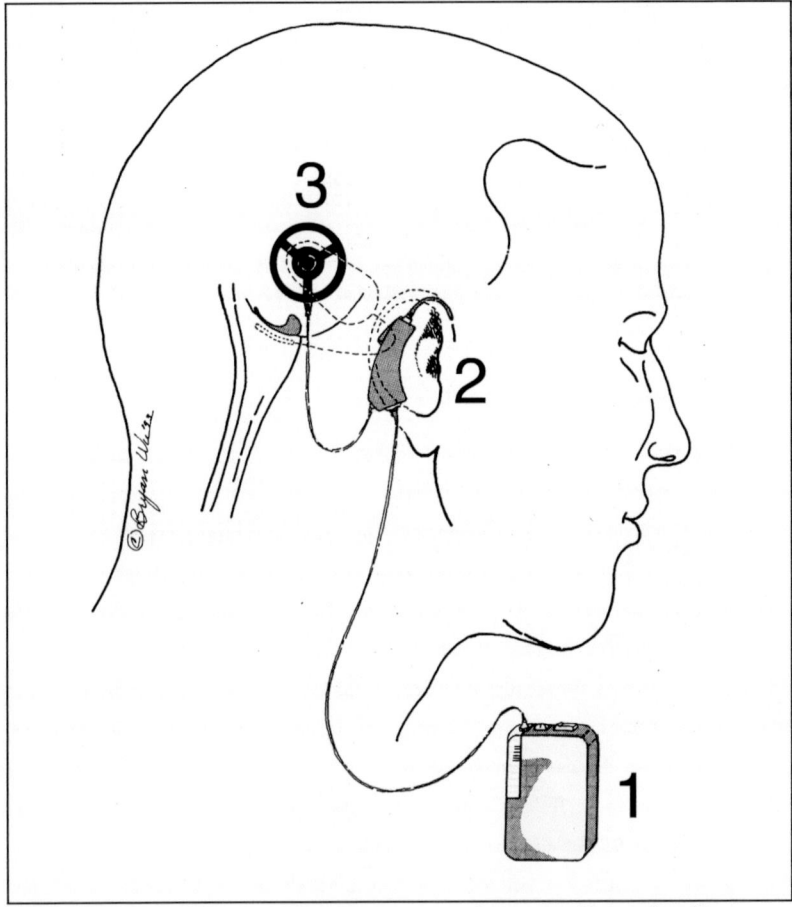

Figure 5: External components of the ABI system: speechprocessor (1), ear-clip with microphone (2) and transmitter coil (3) placed over the implant behind the ear (implanted components see Fig. 6).

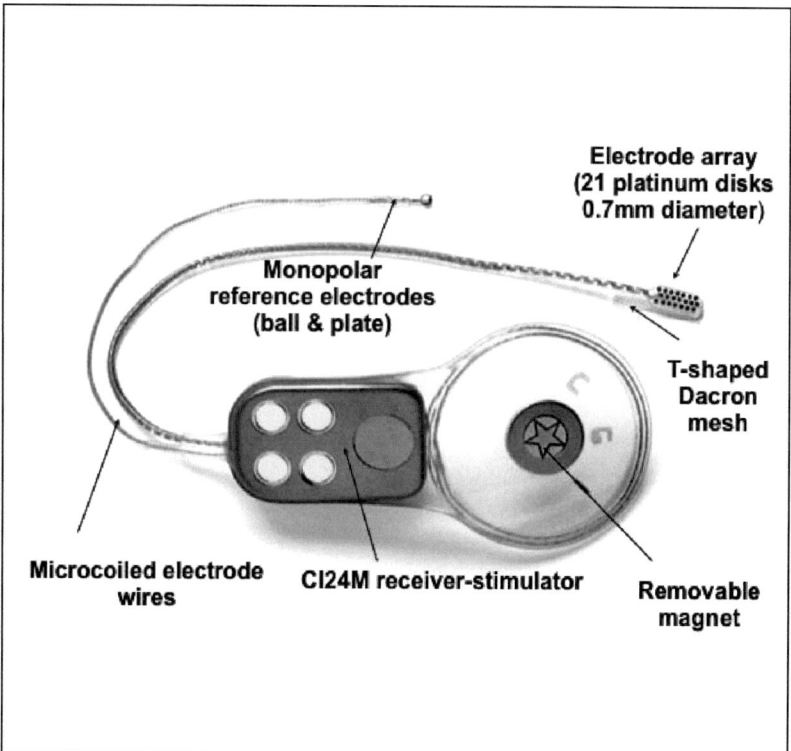

Figure 6: Implanted components of the ABI system: The receiver coil with a removable magnet in center is attached to the receiver/stimulator (R/S) device. The removable magnet helps to keep the external transmitting coil (Component 3 in Figure 5) in place. Since MRI compatibility is markedly improved without the magnet, recently in all patients implanted at HEI, the magnet is removed. The multichannel electrode carrier and a monopolar reference electrode are attached to the other side of the R/S device. The complete R/S device is implanted subcutaneously behind the ear.

1.4.2. Micro- neurosurgical ABI implantation: surgical details

Since minimally invasive implantation of ABI electrodes is not available up to now, the retrosigmoid and the translabyrinthine approach are the microsurgical techniques for electrode placement. Also a subtonsillar ABI placement (Seki et al 2003) via an extended retrosigmoid approach has been described.

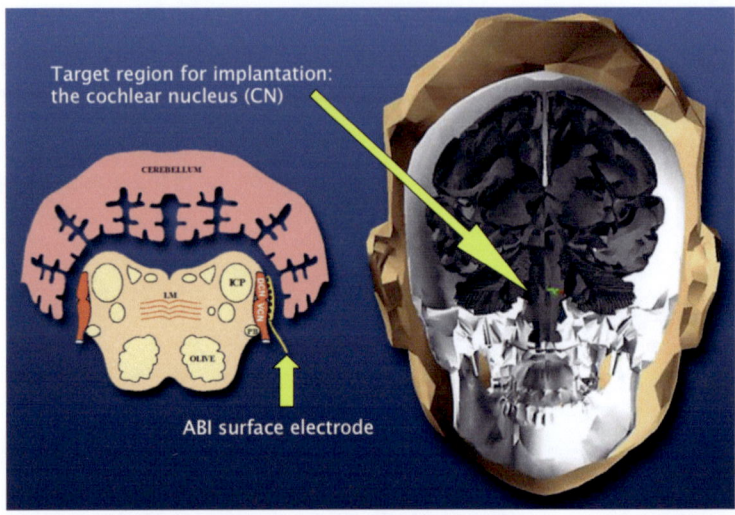

Figure 7: The cochlear nucleus (CN) is the target region for functional ABI stimulation in the brainstem. The image on the right hand side is a three-dimensional reconstruction of individual computer tomography scans. The arrow points to the target area which is located in a region that can be described as the geographical center of the head. The image on the left represents a histologic section through the brainstem at the level of the cochlear nucleus after translabyrinthine dissection and tumor removal. The electrode plate is implanted into the lateral recessus of the 4th ventricle. Non- auditory structures in vicinity to the ventral and dorsal part of the CN (VCN and DCN, axial section on the left side) include the cerebellum, the pontobulbar body (PB) and the inferior cereblellar peduncle (ICP).

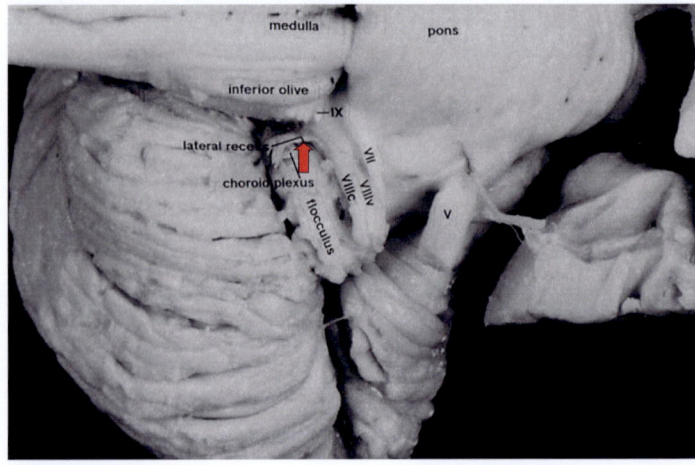

Figure 8 : Anatomical specimen simulating surgical view while implanting the ABI electrode via the translabyrinthine approach. The arrow indicates the entrance into the 4th ventricle. Closeby non-auditory structures include the cranial nerves VII, IV, X and XI, the flocculus, the pontobulbar body (PB) and the inferior cerebellar peduncle (ICP, see also Figure 7). Assuming a theoretical range of stimulation of 1mm/mA, with a maximum ABI current of 2mA, auditory and non-auditory structures within a range of 2mm may be stimulated by the implant. (anatomic specimen photographed in collaboration with the House Ear Institute, Los Angeles, Anatomic Lab, Dr. Fred Linthicum).

The translabyrinthine approach offers a direct angle of view to the lateral recess of the fourth ventricle.   An alternative for ABI placement is the retrosigmoid or lateral suboccipital approach (Colletti et al, 2000). The main argument for use of the retrosigmoid approach is the potential to preserve hearing since the cochlea is not destroyed during the operative approach. Other advantages include a shorter operative times and a reduced risk of cerebrospinal fluid (CSF) leakage. Its disadvantages include difficulty in placing the lead appropriately. Other approaches include the subtonsillar or telovelar approaches via a midline suboccipital craniotomy (Seki et al, 2003) and ABI placement through one of the standard approaches but with endoscope-assisted technique (Friedland et al, 1999).   The advantages of a subtonsillar approach include superior visualization of the floor of the fourth ventricle and the absence of scarring of the surgical corridor.

1.4.3. Speech processor programming

Due to the risk of stimulating the ninth and tenth cranial nerves, the initial testing should be conducted with emergency medical assistance readily available. At the initial stimulation, threshold and comfort levels were measured in monopolar mode (receiver case ground) for each electrode, and comments were elicited from the patient regarding the magnitude of any nonauditory responses as well as the sound quality (especially pitch) of auditory responses. Speech processors for auditory prostheses have a large number of parameters to adjust. Research with cochlear implants has suggested that nonsimultaneous pulses are important for avoiding electrical current field interactions that can occur with simultaneous activation of two or more electrodes. Thus, most present implant speech processors use high-rate nonsimultaneous pulses on multiple electrodes.

Brainstem implant and cochlear implant listeners provide dramatically reduced amplitude ranges. Proper mapping of loudness from acoustic to electrical domains is important for speech recognition in electrical hearing. Several studies have measured speech recognition with custom loudness functions for each electrode (Boex et al., 1997) or under parametric variation in the loudness mapping function (Fu and Shannon, 1998b; Shannon et al., 1992). These studies found that speech recognition was only mildly effected by relatively large variations in the acoustic-to-electrical loudness mapping functions (10-15% decrement in vowel recognition). Thus while the loudness function may contribute to overall quality and naturalness of a speech processor, it appears to be a relatively minor factor in speech recognition performance. There has also been a long-standing discussion about the temporal resolution of hearing-impaired and cochlear implant listeners. The raw psychophysical data indicates that impaired listeners have poorer temporal resolution than unimpaired listeners. However, when the data are plotted in terms of equal loudness, i.e. corrected for the hearing loss, the measures of temporal performance look quite normal. At present, the dominant view is that temporal processing is relatively normal in hearing impaired and implant listeners, once the amplitude is properly mapped to preserve loudness. One factor in the reduced speech recognition ability of hearing-impaired listeners is thought to be poor frequency resolution (as evidenced by wider psychophysical tuning curves). Good spectral selectivity is thought to improve the spectral analysis of the speech signal, allowing finer frequency and formant discrimination. In electrical auditory prostheses the spectral (or tonotopic) resolution is determined by the number of electrodes and by the interaction of those electrodes.

In a patient with poor nerve survival or poor electrode placement, even a large number of electrodes may be so highly interactive that they function as if they were carrying only a single channel of information. Thus, it is important to assess the degree of interaction between electrodes in a cochlear implant and auditory brainstem implant. It is widely assumed that speech recognition should improve as the number of channels of information is increased, although recent data show that there is a point of diminishing returns between 4 and 8 channels (Dorman et al., 1997a; Fishman et al., 1997; Shannon et al., 1995). In more challenging listening conditions, such as in background noise, more channels are necessary to maintain performance at high levels (Delhorne et al., 1997; Fu et al, 1998). Interestingly, cochlear implant listeners appear to utilize only 4-7 channels of information in speech, even though their devices have as many as 20 electrodes, demonstrating that there is not a one-to-one relation between the number of electrodes and the number of channels of usable information. However, considerable open-set speech recognition with cochlear implants is possible with as few as 3-4 channels (Hill et al., 1969; Shannon et al., 1995; Dorman et al., 1997b), so that implant patients are performing well with 4-7 channels, even if this level is sub-optimal relative to the capabilities of the device. To find out how many channels are required to achieve speech recognition in ABI is one of the tasks of the study presented here (chapter 2.13). Daniloff et al., 1968; Nagafuchi, 1976; Tiffany and Bennett, 1961 have shown that spectral information in speech can be shifted by about 60% (about 3 mm in tonotopic coordinates) without serious degradation in intelligibility. However, shifts larger than 60% resulted in large decrements, so that by a shift of an octave speech recognition was almost completely eliminated. Fu and Shannon show almost the same quantitative pattern in cochlear implants and in normal-hearing listeners simulating cochlear implants. The convergence of data from these diverse studies suggests that the alignment of the spectral information in speech with the proper tonotopic location is a critical factor in speech recognition. This is important for the placement and programming of all kinds of possible central auditory implants.

Even if the spectral information is presented to the proper tonotopic location, the homogenity of this mapping can play a major role in speech recognition. Due to the specific pathology leading to deafness of each individual patient, the underlying nerve survival in the areas stimulated might be uneven. This uneven (or nonhomogeneous) nerve survival would distort the uniformity of the mapping between the spectral representation of speech and the pattern of neural activation. Such "holes" in the nerve survival would have the effect of warping the spectral representation. Experiments in the laboratory with cochlear implant listeners and with normal-hearing listeners simulating cochlear implants have shown that this kind of warping can seriously degrade speech recognition (Fu and Shannon, 1998a). In an ABI, such matching of the absolute tonotopic location and spacing is much more difficult because we cannot be certain which tonotopic subunit in the cochlear nucleus we are stimulating. During the postoperative programming of the device it is a very delicate task of the audiologist to measure or estimate the absolute tonotopic location of the ABI electrodes and adjust the speech processor accordingly.

1.4.4. Intraoperative neuromonitoring

Postoperative perceptual performance in ABI is related to correct positioning of the stimulating electrode array in the vicinity of the auditory pathways, i.e. the cochlear nucleus. Since anatomical landmarks are sometimes not easy to identify after the resection of the tumor, the development of intraoperative electrophysiological aids is of great clinical importance. Verification of appropriate electrode placement and system integrity is accomplished through the recording of the Electrical Auditory Brainstem Response, EABR. Neural integrity of the seventh and ninth cranial nerves is also monitored constantly with electromyography throughout the procedure.

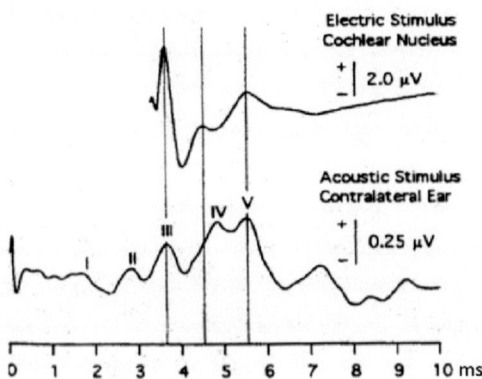

Figure 9: Auditory brainstem responses evoked by electrical stimulation of the cochlear nucleus in human subjects. The upper curve shows the compound action potential in response to electrical stimulation at the cochlear nucleus. The lower curve represents a "conventional" auditory evoked potential with 1000 95 dB rarefaction clicks averaged (from Waring, 1995).

Over the last years the recording of late auditory responses using various electrophysiological techniques have been employed to achieve a better view about the stimulability of the central auditory pathways. Electrically evoked auditory brainstem response (EABR) testing proved to be a helpful intraoperative tool in auditory brainstem implantation (Waring et al, 1995). It has been shown that the intraoperative recording of

EABR is able to confirm the activation of the auditory structures with the implanted ABI system. EABR ´s are most appropriate for this purpose because all longer-latency auditory evoked potentials are more likely to be depressed and unreliable when the patient is anesthetized. One disadvantage of EABR recording is that multiple subdermal needle electrodes have to be placed at the vertex of the head (Cz) and over C7 at the neck. EABR monitoring also requires an additional computer for stimulation and recording of the potentials in the operating room.

1.5.   Penetrating auditory brainstem implants (PABI)

The function of the dorsal cochlear nucleus (DCN) is not well understood. It is thought to have a general alerting function, and possibly some role in sound localization (Masterton, 1992). Unfortunately, the tonotopic axis of the DCN is orthogonal to the axis of the surface electrode array in the "conventional" surface ABI (chapters 1-2). Thus, even if each electrode is stimulating a distinct group of fibers, we might not always expect the electrodes to elicit different pitches. If the limiting factor in ABI performance is that the surface electrode is stimulating the wrong subunit of the CN and/or stimulating in a nontonotopic manner, then a penetrating microelectrode could overcome these problems by stimulating the CN locally and tonotopically. If the limiting factor is that direct electrical stimulation bypasses or interferes with intrinsic neural processing within the CN, then the same limitation might apply to penetrating electrodes. Physiological results with penetrating microelectrodes in the cochlear nucleus of cats (McCreery et al., 1997) have demonstrated a stimulus induced depression of neural excitability (SIDNE). This depression of excitability becomes quite severe at pulse rates of 500 Hz and faster, and the depression can last for many days following termination of stimulation. Although there is presently no evidence of anatomical damage associated with SIDNE, we must prepare to stimulate a penetrating electrode ABI with low rates.Present speech processors utilize nonsimultaneous stimulation on multiple electrodes, with rates of 250 pps to 1000 pps. If SIDNE indicates a stimulation regime that should be avoided, the high pulse rate speech processors would not be suitable for microelectrode stimulation of the cochlear nucleus. However, it is not clear if low pulse rate processors would produce poorer speech recognition than high pulse rate processors. Shannon et al. (1995) showed no significant deterioration in speech recognition when speech envelope information was limited to below 50 Hz.

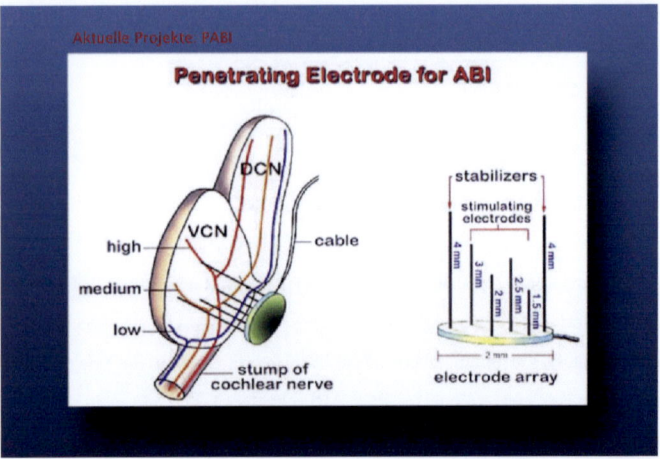

Figure 10: Three-dimensional distribution of frequency layers inside the cochlear nucleus. While the low frequencies are represented at the surface of the CN, the higher frequencies are represented deep within the CN. Penetreating electrodes (PABI) are able to access all frequencies independently. According to my results from section 2.9.2. in this paper, the array should be targeting the ventral nucleus (VCN) rather than the dorsal cochlear nucleus (DCN).

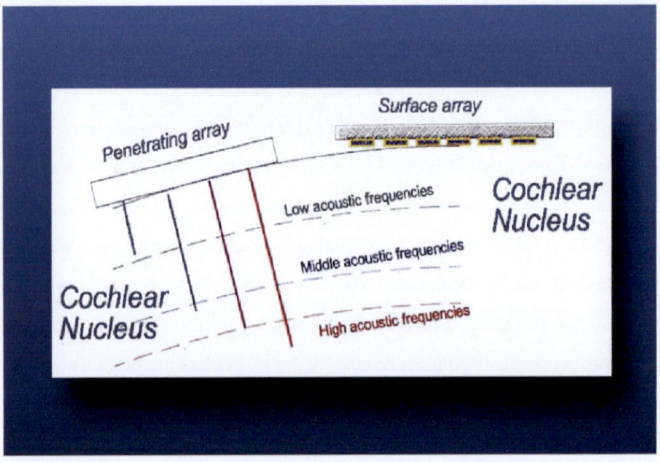

Figure 11: A combination of a PABI electrode and ABI surface electrode implanted in vicinity to the ventral part of the cochlear nucleus (VCN) like performed in the patients reported on in chapter 3.4. Three dimensional frequency layers of the CN with representations of low sounds at the surface and higher frequencies in the deep of the nucleus are displayed. With PABI, the stimulation is no more limited to the surface areas where only the low frequencies are processed. This is the reason why the sound quality of speech is not so much "muffeld" anymore, which makes neuroprosthetic hearing more comfortable.

Because surface electrodes are expected to activate broader tonotopic regions, speech processors have been developed that use surface electrodes for low-frequency information, which can be conveyed primarily temporally, and use the penetrating electrode for higher-frequency spectral information that is conveyed primarily by tonotopic location. The frequency dividing these two spectral ranges is parametrically adjusted to determine the best balance between spectral and temporal representations.

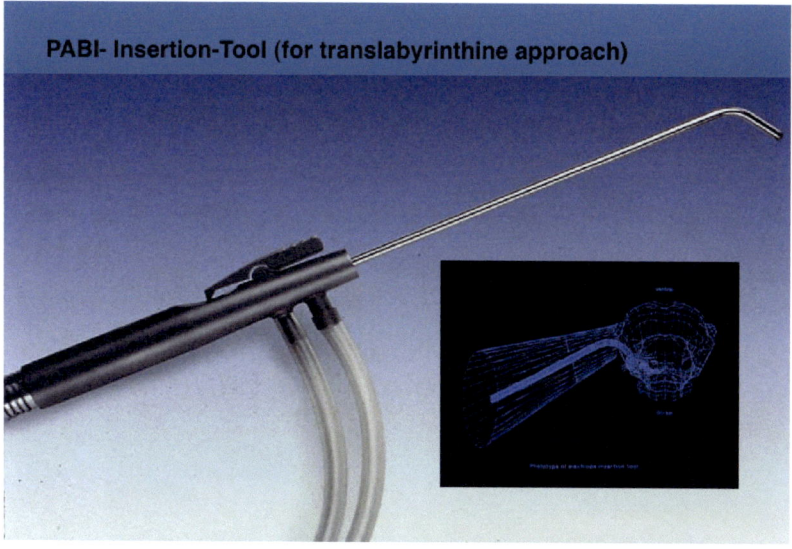

Figure 12: Applicator tool developed at HMRI in collaboration with the Department of Auditory Implants and Perception (DAIP) at HEI. The device is designed to hold the implant without damaging the thin electrode contacts during insertion into the lateral recess. A surgical suction is attached to the device. Pushing the button "shoots" the implant through the glia limitans into the cochlear nucleus. After PABI implantation the applicator is retracted and the surface implant is placed into the lateral recess using a surgical forceps.

Up to now five patients have now received the penetrating auditory brainstem implant (PABI). After resection of vestibular schwannomas, they were implanted with an array of 14 macroelectrodes that resides in the lateral recess over the cochlear nucleus, and an array of 8 activated iridium microelectrodes that penetrate into the nucleus. Penetrating electrodes have produced auditory percepts in three of five patients and produced neither auditory nor non-auditory effects in two patients ("PABI non-stims"). Radiological evidence indicates that the penetrating electrode assembly was dislodged from its implanted location in PABI#4. Radiological results from PABI#5 are pending. No PABI patient is receiving significant open-set speech recognition, even though PABI#1 and #2 have more than one year of experience. The two PABI patients who receive auditory percepts from multiple penetrating electrodes prefer the sound of a "mixed" electrode map, which is comprised of both surface and penetrating electrodes. PABI recipients are typically fitted with three speech processor maps for take-home use: a map that uses only surface electrodes, one that uses only penetrating electrodes (if possible) and a map that uses a combination of surface and penetrating electrodes. They are instructed to try each map to see if one is better suited for different listening conditions than the others. PABI patients 2 and 3, who have multiple functional penetrating electrodes, prefer the combination map for all listening conditions. PABI#1, who has only one penetrating that produces audition, prefers the surface only map. In PABI patients #2 and #3, the map utilizing only penetrating electrodes is usually too soft (due to charge limit of 3 nC/phase) or sounds too mechanical.

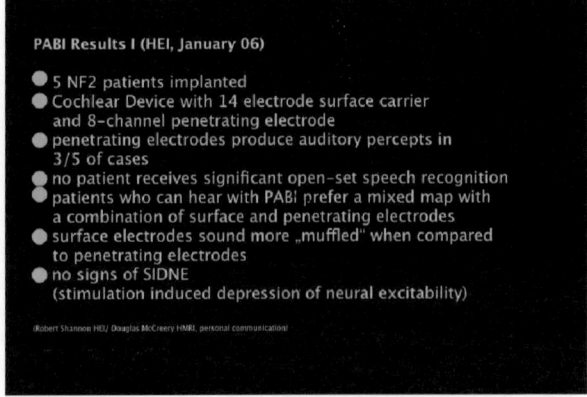

Figure 13: Preliminary PABI results, (Robert Shannon, personal communication)

Results up to now indicate that penetrating deep brain electrode implantation into the central auditory pathways is possible and efficient using the "conventional" otoneurosurgical translabyrinthine approach. Although perceptual performance of the patients up to now is not statistically significant superior to surface electrodes alone, the quality of the speech transmitted by the PABI/ surface ABI combination is subjectively much better when compared to the surface ABI alone. No disadvantages or additional specific complications (see chapter 2.8-2.10) of penetrating ABI implants became evident.

1.6.   Stimulating the inferior colliculus (IC)

Many areas along the auditory pathways represent possible candidates for prosthetic stimulation (please see also Figure 1). In the case of a disconnection of the auditory pathways proximal to the cochlea, the target region of the "common" ABI as reported in the previous chapters is the surface of the cochlear nucleus. As a rule of thumb, the quality of speech perceived with an auditory implant is decreasing, the more central the target of stimulation is. The reason for this is that up to now we have no complete understanding about what happens with the auditory information from the cochlea to the auditory cortex. Thereby we are very far from being able to imitate any of the sound processings that occur along the central auditory pathways.

The inferior colliculus (IC) is a very important central station along the auditory pathway in the midbrain. The IC is an obligatory way station for the transmission of spectral information to the auditory cortical area. Both the VCN and the DCN project to the IC, but the pathway from the VCN is about ten times more voluminous. Sophisticated research has been performed (Schreiner et al) to characterize the response characteristics of the IC to peripheral acoustic or electrical stimulation. The IC appears to be an integrative station as well as a switchboard. A spatio-topic map of the auditory environment has been detected also in response to amplitude differences and interaural delays. The principle of tonotopy is also important in the structure of the IC; different areas of the IC respond differently to different frequencies applied. Anatomically, the IC contains three distinct nuclei when stained in Nissl sections. The different areas of the IC show a different responsibility to specific phonemes and intonations necessary for speech recognition. Important regarding possible side-effects in response to prosthetic stimulation with the SAI is that the IC seems also to be involved with several more complex functions. Cat experiments have shown that also the startle reflex and ocular reflexes are influenced by activity in the IC, although this does not necessarily prove non-auditory effects since this reflex modulation can also occur with auditory stimulation. The tuning curves in the IC exhibit a complexity beyond that found at lower levels of the brainstem. The IC is tonotopically arranged in isofrequency (same center frequency) stripes with running dorso-caudal to ventro-rostral. These stripes roughly correspond with the tracts of axons entering the IC from the lateral lemniscus. Interestingly, the sharpness of the tuning curves found within an isofrequency stripe is not uniform. Instead, cells with the sharpest tuning curves seem to be located in the center of the IC, while cells with progressively broader tuning curves are arranged in concentric bands.

Cells in the IC vary their responses in proportion to several parameters besides intensity and frequency including phase, intensity and the bandwidth of a stimulus. Cells have been found in the IC which are maximally responsive to a specific frequency of amplitude modulation of a pure tone. Binaural interactions appear to be prominent in the ICC as well. One type of cell, the EE type, responds to a characteristic temporal delay. In contrast to similar EE cells in the SOC, these cells have very broad tuning curves making their responses relatively independent of frequency. They also respond continuously when a sound source located at a specific azimuth or angle in relation to the head. The response seems to be maximal when the sound source is located on the contralateral side of the head from the responding ICC. Another cell type, the EI, responds best when the amplitude of a sound is louder in the contralateral than the ipsilateral ear. Thus, the ability to localize the angle at which a sound source is located becomes more generalized at the level of the IC. Again, no reports about experiments with stimulation of the IC and recording at higher levels of the auditory system have been reported before 2001 (please see following chapter). Concerning the implantation of NF2 patients or other lesions of the 8th nerve, one advantage of stimulating the IC is that it is not affected by the primary deafening lesion.

1.6.1. Stereotactic deep brain implantation

Stereotactic neurosurgery has become an indispensible portion of the neurosurgical repertoire, a method allowing three dimensional localization of specific sites within the nervous system. The word stereotactic is derived from Greek word "stereos", meaning "three dimensional", and the Latin word "tactus", meaning "to touch". In the 1940s, physicians attempted to treat parkinsons disease by creating defects within selected brain areas associated with movement disorders. Stereotactic guidance was used to increase the accuracy of the lesion produced. In the last 30 years, imaging techniques like CT and MRI redefined the ability of physicians to identify and locate diseases within the brain. The initial step to stereotactic localization until today is the application of a fixed head ring (frameless techniques have been developed which are under clinical investigation). A localizing ring is attached to the head holder and imaging is performed with the head fixed inside the ring. The image obtained allows the neurosurgeon to compute the exact three dimensional target inside the region of interest. A small incision is made at the entry side and a hole is drilled through the skull. The needle/ electrode is inserted through a guiding cannula to the point of interest inside the brain. The operation can be performed under local anaesthesia with the patient fully awake and responsible. Stereotactic deep brain electrode implantation was approved by the Federal Drug Administration (FDA) in the US for the treatment of tremor (target region: ventro intermediate nucleus of the thalamus (Deuschl and Bain, 2002)) and parkinsons disease (target region: subthalamic nucleus, (Pollack et al 2002)). Experimental studies were undertaken for epilepsy (Hamani and Hodaie, 2002), chronic pain (Kumar et al 1997), dystonia (Vercueil et al 2002), apallic syndrome (Yamamoto et all 2002) and coma (Sturm et al 1979). Since 1995 deep brain implantation is approved for the treatment of tremor in parkinsons disease also in Germany. Until the end of 2002 more than 20000 patients were treated worldwide with deep brain electrodes (Medtronic company, Düsseldorf 2003). Reported sucess rates for the reduction of tremor, akinesia and rigor in parkinosons disease are above 80% (Benabid et al 2003). One big advantage of deep brain stimulation when compared to ablative techniques is its reversibility. Other advantages are the low rate of side-effects when compared to the common lesional techniques. Electrode implantation and stimulation do not cause functionally relevant brain damage. The stimulating current can be switched off or modified when unwanted side-effects occur.

1.6.2. Stereotactic Neurosurgery in Cologne

The Department of Stereotaxy and Functional Neurosurgery at Cologne University is one of
the most experienced centers of this kind in the world. The chairman (Volker Sturm) holds the
only academic chair for Stereotactic Neurosurgery in Germany. The Department of Stereotaxy
at Cologne University has three operating theaters, two of which are equipped with
conventional X-ray systems for localization. The third operating room incorporates a 1.5 Tesla
MRI as well as sophisticated hard-and software for target localization and the planning of the
approach. The 1.5 Tesla MRI allows intraoperative functional neuroimaging. With more than
220 patients threated with bilateral subthalamic nucleus electrode implantation for parkinsons
disease, it is the center with the biggest series of this kind in the world. Experience with deep-
brain electrode implantation over many years as well as optimal technical and personal
conditions (a team of 4 full-time specialized engeneers to assist with the planning of the
stereotactic approaches) resulted in a reduction of intraoperative hermorrhagic complications
from 1.5% to 0.6% today.

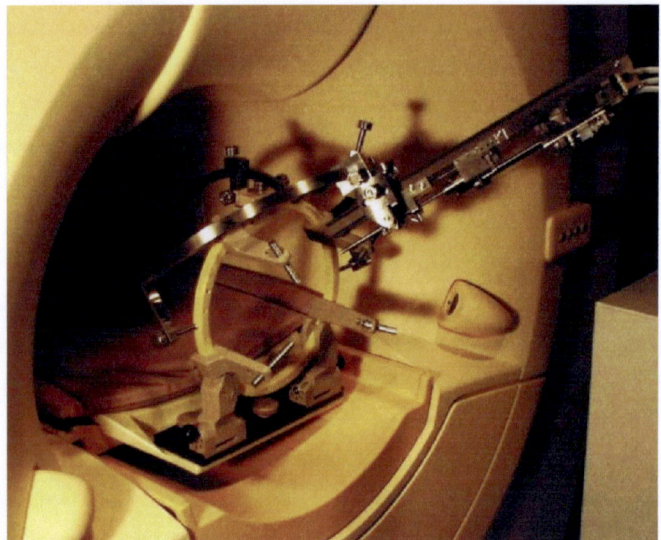

Figure 14: Computer assisted stereotactic guiding system and intraoperative MRI
(Department of Stereotaxy and Functional Neurosurgery, Cologne University, Cologne,
Germany)

2.   Methods

2.1.   Retrospective ABI study: Data analysis

2.1.1.   Speech perception with auditory brainstem implants

Until 2001, no database existed at HEI containing preoperative, intraoperative, radiological and audiological data of the implanted patients. The first step as research fellow was to implement a   SPSS 11.0 database and aquire all available data of the ABI patients. Postoperative imaging (MRI/ CT) was not performed in most patients. In February 2001, all implanted ABI patients were contacted for the purpose of this study and asked to perform a postoperative MRI or CT scan to evaluate the position of the implanted device. All available audiological data from the patients (side effects and audiological test-results in relation to stimulation parameters in 347 postoperative testing and programming sessions) was enclosed into this new database. The postoperative clinical follow-up included audiological examinations with clinical testing and/ or reprogramming of the devices at 6 weeks, 3 months, 6 months, 9 months and 12 months in the first year and at least once a year in the further postoperative course. All audiologic tests were performed by the same audiologist (S.O.).

Postoperatively all electrodes were tested routinely in monopolar mode to measure individual threshold and comfort levels. Perceptual performance was tested using tests for sound effect recognition (SERT), vowel and consonant recognition, word and word-stress recognition (MTS), sentence recognition (NUCHIPS and CUNY). Sixty-one patients with neurofibromatosis Type 2 (NF2) received the Nucleus 8 electrode multi-channel ABI implant (Cochlear Corperation, Englewood, CO) at the House Ear Institute/ Los Angeles between September 1992 and December 1999. The Nucleus ABI uses the Spectra sound processor with the SPEAK (spectral maxima) processing strategy (McDermott, 1992). Patients were tested and programmed initially about six weeks postoperatively and every 3 months in the first year thereafter. Threshold and comfort levels were measured in monopolar mode (receiver case ground) for each electrode, and non-auditory side-effects (NASE) were ranked on a visual analog scale ranging from 0-4 with grade 1=slightly noticeable and 4=severe/ intolerable. Perceptual performance was assessed at every follow up interval by an extensive test battery including the Sound-Effects Recognition Test (SERT), the Iowa Consonant and

Vowel test, the MTS (Monosyllable Trochee Spondee) test, the Children's Perception of Speech Test (NU-CHIPS), and the City University of New York (CUNY) sentence recognition test.

The SERT test is a four-alternative test of environmental sound discrimination with chance performance level of 25%. These sounds were not matched in their temporal patterns or frequency content so that identification of their temporal patterns could allow correct identification. The vowel, consonant and CUNY sentence tests were all presented in sound-only, vision-only and sound-plus-vision modes. All other tests were administered in sound-only mode. For the purpose of this study only the sound only results were evaluated. A single male talker produced both vowels and consonants. Constant confusion matrices were compiled from five presentations of 16 medial consonants (ama, ana, afa, etc.) for each listener. Vowel confusions matrices were compiled from three presentations of 8 vowels in a h/V/d context (heed, hid, had, etc.). Chance performance level of the consonant recognition test was 7.14% correct and the 95% confidence level was 11.1% correct. ABI recipients with no residual hearing were tested in a standard fashion seated 1 meter in front of a loudspeaker with test items presented at 60dB hearing level and processors adjusted for comfortable loudness. Patients implanted on their first-tumor sides who had some remaining hearing on their second-tumor sides were tested through an audio interface (Nucleus) with the loudspeaker bypassed and sounds delivered directly to the audio input of the sound processor. During the initial fitting session, the subjective pitch of the auditory percepts on each useable electrode was assessed on a visual analog scale ranging from 1 (lowest pitch) to 100 (highest pitch). Ten judgements were obtained per electrode, which yielded an estimate of the range and variability of pitch percepts and suggested the degree to which electrodes may have been activating different neural populations. The overall pitch range was defined as the range from the lowest to the highest subjective pitch sensation on the visual analog scale (1-100, chapter 2.7.). When all stimulated channels had the same pitch, or the patient was unable to assess the pitch level, the overall pitch range was 0. For statistical analysis, test results and electrode "maps" were analysed and the relations between the different conditions were evaluated using the paired T-test and repeated measures ANOVA.

During the first postoperative programming pitch rank of electrically evoked auditory sensations was assessed using a visual analogue scale ranging from 0 to 100. On the base of this frequency allocation tables and the determined C-and T-levels an individual matching map was created for every patient. Patients were split in two groups a) having an interelectrode pitch magnitude range of 30 or more units and group b) having an interelectrode pitch magnitude range of less than 30 units through the array. The performance of group a and b was analysed separately in terms of vowel, consonant, and open speech recognition. The number of auditory and non-auditory electrodes was determined in both groups. Non-auditory side-effects (NASE) were assessed by type (spasm, contraction, jitter, tingling, vibration etc.), location (eye, ear, mouth, etc.) and by lateralization in relation to the implant (ipsilateral / contralateral / bilateral). During all postoperative consultations the ranking of the magnitude of the side-effects was assessed on a visual analog scale from 0-4 (0=none, 1=notice slightly, 2=present consistently but tolerable, 3=unpleasant, 4=intolerable).

2.1.2. The number of functional electrodes in auditory brainstem implants

Speech perception is dependent on the recognition of both spectral and temporal cues. There has been an intensive and fruitful discussion in recent years regarding how many individual channels are necessary to achieve good consonant and vowel recognition. Though a limited degree of consonant recognition is possible even in the absence of spectral cues (Van Tasell et al., 1992; Van Tasell et al., 1987), a significant intra-individual improvement of perceptual performance has been demonstrated from single-channel to multi-channel electrodes in cochlear implant recipients. (Dorman et al., 1989, 1997b; Fishman et al., 1997).

In order to investigate these relations in normal listeners, modulated noise bands were used to simulate the different spectral channels in a cochlear implant speech processor (Shannon et al., 1995) . The temporal envelope of the speech signal was extracted from different frequency bands and used to modulate a noise signal. High levels of speech performance were obtained in normal listeners with as few as four spectral bands. Shannon et al. also found that it is important to match the frequency band of the coded speech information with the delivered noise carrier band and in frequency location. Severe mismatch in cochlear implants presents the information to an inappropriate location on the cochlea, thereby limiting auditory performance. This "warping" in the tonotopic dimension significantly impedes the use of spectral information. As in cochlear implantation, the performance of ABI recipients also varies depending on the way the system is programmed (Otto et al., 1998). Not all implanted electrodes provide pure auditory sensations, and so most patients can use only a portion of the implanted electrodes on the carrier. The purpose of this study was to document and analyse how the perceptual performance in these multi-electrode ABI systems varies in relation to the number of functional auditory electrodes on their Nucleus 8-channel surface array. Audiological tests were performed acccording to the technique described in the previous chapter.

2.1.3. Auditory brainstem implantation after previous radiosurgery

A retrospective analysis was performed in 132 patients with NF 2 who received auditory brainstem implants between 1997 and 2001 at the House Ear Institute (HEI), USA. Magnetic resonance tomographic images were reviewed for detectable radiosurgical defects. Operation reports and postoperative audiological findings were reviewed to assess the outcome of ABI with previous radiosurgery.

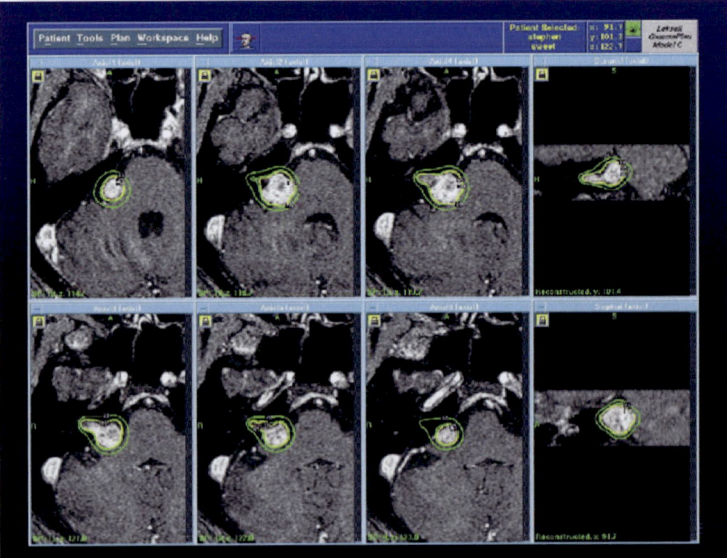

Figure 15: Stereotactic convergent beam irradiation plan (CBI) in a patient with a vestibular schwannoma in the right CPA.

2.2.   Imaging study

2.2.1. Postoperative electrode positions: The electrode-brain interface

After contacting the implanted ABI patients, postoperative imaging data was available from 58 out of the 119 implanted patients. For this retrospective study, the postoperative position of the implanted electrodes was examined on the basis of gradient-echo MRI or edge-enhanced CCT scans. Radiologic findings of the implanted electrodes were correlated to the audiologic results. The radiologic images were reviewed independently by a radiologist (W.L.), a neurosurgeon (J.K.) and an otologist (J.F.). The position of the electrode array was classified by each observer. Cases were excluded from further evaluation if there was inter-individual disagreement about the electrode postion relative to the lateral recess and cochlear nucleus region. Categories of ABI positions in relation to the CN were defined in collaboration with Jane Moore, Ph.D., Dep. of Neuroanatomy, HEI, 2001, see appendix page 124).

The position of the ABI electrode at the surface of the cochlear nucleus is an important factor for the clinical outcome. One issue of concern has been the possibility that a shift in position of the brainstem after removal of the tumor mass would cause a change in the electrode position relative to the targeted brainstem structures. Over time, a fibrous connective tissue capsule forms around the electrode array. A fibrotic capsule was observed surrounding and infiltrating an electrode array that was removed from one of the early patients 22 months after implantation (Terr et al, 1989). Histologic examination of the capsule indicated that it was fibroblastic in nature and highly invasive of the Dacron mesh carrier. It is not known how much time is required for such a capsule to form in patients; heavy connective tissue ingrowth of Dacron mesh carriers occurs in experimental animals within 2 weeks of implantation. Intraoperative documentation included the size of the lateral recess which was estimated on a visual analogue scale between "small (1)" and „huge (4) by the implanting surgeon (W.H.).

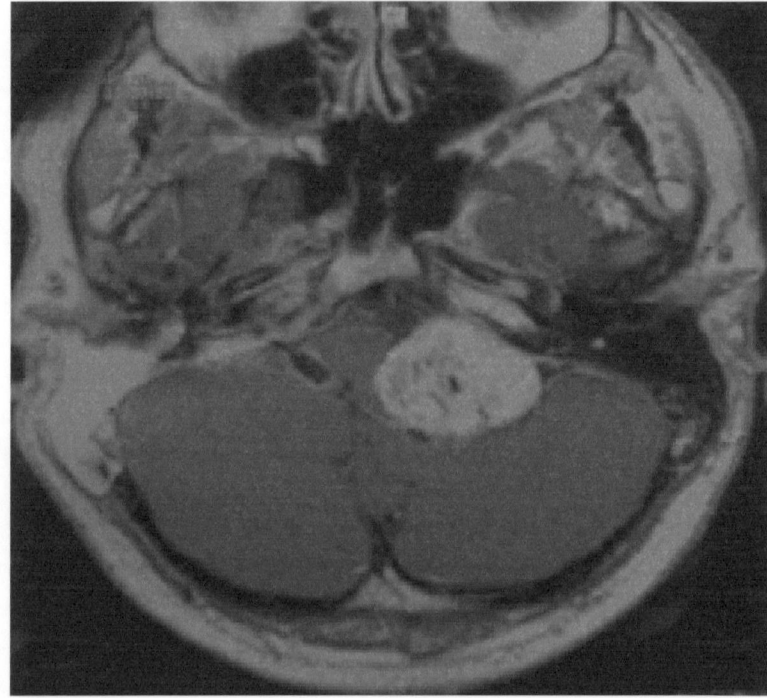

Figure 16: MRI of the cerebellopontine angle in a patient with NF2. A nucleus-24 multi-channel brainstem implant was brought into the lateral recessus of the 4th ventricle at the left side of the picture. The electrode carrier is slightly rotated so that the individual electrodes which are in contact to the surface of the cochlear nucleus become visible. On the right side (contralateral) in the picture there is still a large contrast enhancing tumor compressing the brainstem which will be removed in a second operation.

2.3.   Intraoperative electrophysiological studies

2.3.1. Neural response telemetry (NRT)

In this chapter the methodologies and applications of a new technique for intraoperative monitoring called neural response telemetry (NRT) will be described. NRT was developed based on the intracochlear measurement of compound action potentials (CAP) used by Brown et al 1990 and is implemented in the Nucleus CI24 auditory brainstem implant system. Due to the proximity of the recording electrodes to the neural structures in the CN, the susceptibility of the signal to noise is considerably better when compared to EABR measurements. For the same reason also the amount of averaging and recording time required to obtain a clear recording is reduced. Postoperative NRT measurements can be conducted with an awake subject who may be reading or moving around. NRT is now used widely for cochlear implant monitoring in more than 200 cases but has not been applied for ABI implantation up to now (Brown et al 1990, Dillier et al 2002).

The intraoperative use of NRT in auditory brainstem implants was evaluated for the first time in a prospective clinical study. The establishment of clear criteria for identifying electrically evoked compound action potentials is a precondition for any clinical application of NRT (see also chapter 4.3.2.: "A new classification of NRT responses in ABI").

Figure 17: Neural response telemetry: "Screenshot" of the NRT software window for selecting the parameters for stimulation, recording, masking and averaging. In this bi-directional telemetric system, radio-frequency pulses are transmitted from the speech processor interface across the skin barrier to the implanted R/S device. The responses to stimulation were averaged, analyzed and the resultant CAP waveform then is displayed on the computer. No additional surface electrodes are necessary.

Because of the non-specific nature of the electrical stimulus, a variety of closeby non-auditory structures may be activated and contaminate the recorded CAP. Of the several sources of signal contamination, stimulus artifact is the most readily identified. Care in minimizing the artifact by proper adjustment of stimulating and recording instrumentation is essential for successful NRT measurement. The most likely sites of non-auditory activation are the facial and vestibular nucleus. It is important to recognize that the evoked potential can be severely contaminated with non-auditory signals long before muscular contractions or EMG changes occur. From 1979 to 2001, 121 patients who became deafened due to vestibular schwannoma (VS) growth received an auditory brainstem implant (ABI) at the House Ear Clinic, Los Angeles.

Standard cranial nerve monitoring and electrically evoked auditory brainstem response (EABR) monitoring was performed to assist electrode placement. In addition to this we (J.K./ S.O.) performed intraoperative NRT using the commercially available windows based NRT v2.04 software installed on a laptop computer in the recent 8 implantations. The Nucleus 24 ABI electrode carrier (Cochelar company, Melblurne, Australia) has 21 distinct stimulation sites. With this system it is possible to stimulate on one location at the surface of the cochlear nucleus and to record the resulting electrically evoked compound action potential (ECAP) from a neighbouring location. By examining various aspects of the response waveform systematically, it may be possible to deduce useful information about the central auditory pathways stimulated. For instance, the size of the response amplitude could be related to the population density of the responding neurons, or their temporal response properties could be related to the capacity of these nerve fibers to transmit information encoded in the rate of stimulation. This capacity of the stimulated neurons in the cochlear nucleus to transmit the electrically encoded information centrally along the auditory pathways is the most critical factor determining the outcome of auditory brainstem implants. With NRT compound actions potentials (CAP's) can be evoked and recorded from the surface of the cochlear nucleus or any other neural structure via a bi-directional radio-frequency link. The NRT software communicates with the IF5 interface card in the PC which, in turn, communicates with machine language control software in the SP5 (SPrint) speech processor, which is in bi-directional wireless communication with the CI24M implant. NRT can export neural response data in a format that can be used by commonly available spreadsheet and graphic software applications. Measurements of EAP morphology, growth, and refractory recovery functions can be obtained intraoperatively as well as postoperatively.

Each of the 21 electrodes of the implanted carrier array (Figure 11) can be coupled to the amplifier in bipolar or monopolar (electrode to MP1/ ground) mode and the compound action potential then measured as the response to a proceeding stimulus. The measured potential is sent telemetrically to the fitting station and to a computer for display, storage and analysis of the waveforms. A critical technical problem of NRT recordings is the ratio between the small amplitude of the compound action potential in comparison to the huge potential of the stimulus artefact. NRT recordings are highly susceptible to contamination by stimulus artifact and by elicted potentials

arising from neighbouring non-auditory structures. The Nucleus and the Clarion HiRes 90k (Advanced Bionics company, Sylmar, CA, USA) systems try to overcome this problem by different concepts: in the nucleus system a three staged blanking amplifier with low internal noise and fast recovery time is used whereas for the clarion system an amplifier was developed with low noise, wide dynamic range and very short recovery time. The Nucleus ABI that was implanted in all cases uses the Spectra sound processor with the SPEAK (spectral maxima) processing strategy. Radio frequency pulses are transmitted from the speech processor interface across the skin barrier to the implanted electronic components. This radio frequency code sequence controls the parameters of stimulation used to evoke the CAP. To measure the CAP, a second series of radio frequency pulses is generated, in which information about the magnitude of the voltage recorded on individual electrodes within the CN at specific times after stimulation is coded and transmitted back out to the speech processor interface. These voltages are averaged and analysed, and the resultant CAP waveform then is displayed on the computer. No surface recording electrodes are necessary. To isolate the relatively small neural action potentials from the stimulus artifact, the NRT software uses a forward masking artefact subtraction paradigm. This technique is a modified version of the method described by Brown et al 1990 for cochlear implant users. Responses are recorded sequentially in two different stimulation conditions. First, a recording is made using a single biphasic current pulse or "probe". The response that is recorded in this stimulus condition consists of the resulting stimulus artifact and the much smaller neural response to the probe (CAP). Typically, the associated small, biological neural response is disguised by the large stimulus. A second recording then is made using a pair of biphasic current pulses. The first pulse in the two-pulse sequence is referred to as the "masker" and the second pulse as the "probe". A short inter-pulse interval (IPI) separates the masker and the probe pulses. When two supra-threshold stimulus pulses are presented separated by a short IPI, the auditory nerve responds to the first pulse of the sequence (masker) and then is refractory at the time that the second current pulse (probe) is presented. Consequently, the recording that is made in the masker-plus-probe condition consists of the probe stimulus artefact without the overlying EAP. A sufficiently long delay is necessary to avoid nonlinear behaviour due to saturation of the amplifier caused by the stimulus artefact. If the delay is too long, important features of the neural response such as a possible first negative peak may be missed. Since this parameter is critical, various delay times in awake implanted ABI patients were tested. With a delay time of 40-50 ms optimal response amplitudes were obtained with minimal distortion due to amplifier saturation and maximum preservation of the early components. Both stimulation and recording can be performed in either monopolar or bipolar configuration. Two protocols, a monopolar configuration using a subcutaneous reference ball electrode (MP1) (Figure 12a) and a bipolar configuration (Figure 12b) were used intraoperatively. Biphasic stimuli of 25us per phase were used for both masker and probe stimuli.

After tumor removal, the entrance to the lateral recess was identified and the electrode carrier was implanted into the assumed position close to the cochlear nucleus. Anatomical landmarks were classified as "easy identifiable" by the surgeon (W.H.) in 7 out of 7 cases. EABR monitoring was also performed first all over the array and then in six different locations in order to obtain a geographical mapping. Response characteristics of each stimulated electrode were communicated to the surgeon and the electrode carryer was shifted into the direction of the clear responses. When the definite position of the electrodes was reached, the external coil of the stimulator device was attached to the computer with the NRT device. NRT recordings were performed from the same electrode combinations used for EABR recordings (Figure 11).

2.4. Laboratory studies

2.4.1. Cadaver study: Implantation and MRI- imaging of a prototype PABI electrode

The surface auditory brainstem implant restores some hearing in more than 200 patients worldwide who have lost hearing due to hearing loss due to growth of vestibular schwannoma (VS) growth. With the aim of accessing the tonotopy and thereby improving the auditory outcome a new penetrating electrode for the cochlear nucleus (CN) has been developed in a collaboration between the House Ear Institute and the Huntington Memorial Institute Pasadena. We (J.K. and W.H.) implanted the new designed penetrating electrode into the CN of a formalin fixed cadaver head using the translabyrinthine approach. Like it was planned in the first PABI patients (Figure 45, p83), we also implanted a FDA-approved surface electrode on the same side. Postoperatively I performed neuroradiologic imaging using 1mm sliced axial CT scans as well as axial and coronar MRI reconstructions (scout, T2, TSE AX, FLAIR, HEMO AX, T2 3D, T2 haste cor thin).

Via a postauricular incision a mastoidectomy was carried out with exposure of the middle fossa plate, the sinodural angle, the sigmoid sinus, the posterior fossa dura and the semicircular canals. The sigmoid sinus was uncovered to allow extradural retraction with a surgical irrigator. A labyrinthectomy was carried out and the facial nerve was identified by locating the vertical crest (Bill's'bar) in the internal auditory canal. After this the posterior fossa dura was opened, exposing the tumor and the cerebellopontine angle (CPA). A plane was developed between the proximal portion of the cochlear nerve and the choroid plexus. The cochlear nerve was followed medially as it enters the lateral recess of the fourth ventricle. The taenia of the fourth ventricle was elevated and the device was placed into the lateral recess over the surface of the dorsal and ventral cochlear nuclei. The two cochlear nuclei lie dorsal lateral (dorsal cochlear nucleus) and ventral lateral (ventral cochlear nucleus) to the inferior cerebellar peduncle at the rostral pole of the medulla. The cell groups related to the vestibular division of C.N. VIII are located more medial to the inferior cerebellar peduncle in the brainstem. To achieve electrical stimulation of this area the surface electrode array is placed in the lateral recess of the fourth ventricle after removal of the VS. The choroid plexus and the taenia serve as landmarks for the opening of the lateral recess.

2.4.2. Animal study: Implantation and stimulation of the IC in cats

As a precondition for the development of a clinically applicable SAI electrode, I have conducted laboratory experiments in July 2001 at the Epstein Laboratory of the University of California at San Francisco (UCSF) and at the Neurophysiological Lab at Huntington Memorial Hospital, Pasadena, CA. After intensive contact via email, the two main specialists regarding central microelectrodes and the inferior colliculus were motivated to participate in this experiment. Participating in this acute animal study were Douglas McCreery , Ph.D., Director of the Neural Engineering Program from the Huntington Memorial Research Institute, Pasadena and Christof Schreiner, M.D., Ph.D. Keck Center for Integrative Neuroscience, University of California at San Francisco (UCSF). The aim of this key experiment was to demonstrate for the first time that with stimulation of the IC, low threshold responses could be recorded in the cortex of a cat thereby providing a basis for possible speech recognition with central auditory implants and clinical stimulation at the level of the IC. Experiments were performed in accordance with the policies of the UCSF concerning animal experiments.

The cat was anesthezized with intramuscular injection of ketamine hydrochloride (45 mg/kg). After shaving of the head, a right-sided trephination was performed. The auditory cortex was exposed. The stimulation electrode was aligned along the tonotopic axis of the IC after performing a   lateral supracerebellar infratentorial approach. According to studies of Schreiner et al, 1997, the individual frequency laminae within the IC have a thickness of around 200um.

The tested impedance of the electrode was 10-20 ohms. The stimulating electrode used for this experiment was provided by Douglas McCreery and is essencially the same type as used for central stimulation with the central penetrating auditory brainstem implant (PABI) described earlier (Figure 11, page 24). The Iridium stimulating microelectrode used for stimulation was fabricated from lenghts of pure iridium wire, 70 um in diameter. A Teflon-insulted lead wire was welded to one end of the iridium shaft, and the other end was shaped to a conical taper by electrolytic etching. The microelectrode has relatively blunt tips (a radius of curvature of approximately 6 um) to reduce tissue injury during insertion into the IC. The entire shaft and wire junction was coated with three thin layers of Epoxylite 6001-50 heat-cured electrode varnish. The insulation was removed from the tip with an erbium laser, leaving a geometric surface area of 1000+- 200 um. The individual electrodes are assembled into an integrated array of four microelectrodes spaced approximately 400 um apart. Electrical stimuli were generated by a signal processing computer and converted to an analogue signal by a 16 bit D/A converter running at a 60-Khz sampling rate. A low impedance attenuator was used to control the stimulation current in a range between 1 an 30 mA. Electrical stimuli consited of capacitively coupled, charge balanced, biphasic square wave pulses of 200 us/ phase with an interstimulus interval of 500ms. This technique was developed by Chris Schreiner at the Epstein Laboratory, UCSF, San Francisco for stimulation of the cochlear nucleus, but was never tested for CI stimulation up to now. A silicon-substrate electrode array (McCreery et al, HMRI) was used for cortical recording of electrically evoked potentials. The recorded signals were filtered with analog DC-blocking and anti-aliasing filters from 2-10 KHz.

2.4.3. Engineering: Development of a prototype stereotactic auditory deep brain electrode

After coming back from L.A. in the beginning of 2002, I was looking for a manufacturer of auditory electrodes who is open to new concepts and ideas. The most experienced company of this kind in Europe is the Med-El company in Innsbruck/ Austria. Because the development of a new electrode and maybe a complete stimulating system altogether would require a close contact with regular personal meetings addressing a company in Europe seemed advantageous. Following an invitation of Prof. Hochmayr (CEO of MedEl), a presentation was given in Innsbruck concerning the concept of stereotactic implantation of a central auditory implant. MedEl agreed to assist in developing and manufacturing a prototype electrode according to my plans and scematic drawings. In return, MedEl would have the primary and exclusive right to produce and sell the system, if a clinical stage of the project is reached in the future. Since the clinical implantation will be performed through a small burr hole and through functional brain tissue, the diameter of the electrode has to be very small, i.e. below 2mm. This excludes every type of plate electrodes as known from the conventrional ABI surface electrodes. A needle-type electrode can easily pass through a stereotactic guiding system as used for deep brain electrode implantation in parkinsons disease. Claude Jolly,

Ph.D, director of electrode development at MedEl was assigned to work with the SAI project. Dr. Jolly was invited to visit the Department of Stereotaxy and Functional Neurosurgery in Cologne and he became familiar with the technique of stereotactic deep brain implantation. The intended design of the electrode carrier was be a hybrid between the MedEl surface ABI electrodes and the Medtronic deep brain electrodes. To provide speech recognition, the new electrode should have at least 8 independently stimulable electrodes like the MedEl electrode (not only four like the Medtronic system) and connect to the existing ABI receiver/ stimulating device. Various arrangements of ring and platelet electrodes on the needle-type carrier are possible. At the end of 2003, two prototypes have been manufactured according to my drawings by Claude Jolly for further laboratory and clinical testing (chapter 3.4.3).

2.4.4. MRI- based stereotactic approach for IC implantation

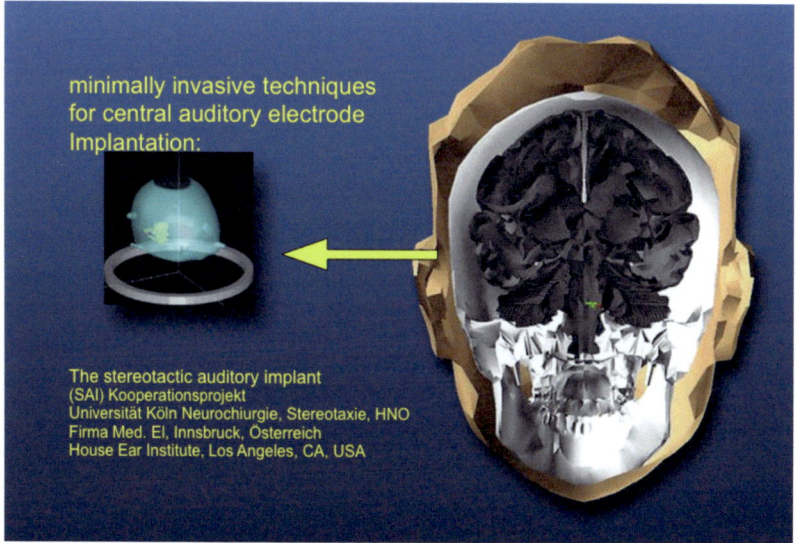

Figure 18: The interdisciplinary multicenter project "Minimally invasive techniques for central auditory electrode implantation, (SAI) was initiated by J.K. in 2003. Participating partners include the Departments of General Neurosurgery, Stereotaxy, ENT (Cologne University), Med-El Company (Innsbruck, Austria) and the Department of Auditory Implants and Perception at the House Ear Institute, Los Angeles, USA.

The supracerebellar infratentorial approach is the choice when targeting the Inferior Colliculus via an open neurosurgical operation. The supracerebellar infratentorial approach provides good exposure of the dorsolateral aspect of the tentorial hiatus and mesencephalon. This approach does not endanger the trochlear nerve or any major midline venous structures in the quadrigeminal cistern. The median infratentorial-supracerebellar route provides direct exposure of the posterior incisural space, although the culmen represents a relative obstacle to exposure of the lower quadrigeminal plate. The paramedian variant allows a more lateral perspective on the posterolateral brainstem surface at the level of the middle incisural space, in addition to exposing the homolateral collicular plate.

The extreme-lateral corridor widens the exposure of the paramedian approach to include the anterolateral brainstem surface, offering a complete view of the cisternal space surrounding the middle incisural space. Nevertheless, for a stereotactic approach and the burr-hole implantation of a needle-type electrode, the requirements are different. The penetrating electrode array has to end up aligned along the well-defined tonotopic gradient of the IC. Although the route from posterior as described above is the shortest, it carries some disadvantages: The electrode has to pass different media, namely the CSF-filled cisterns-therby maybe representing a factor contributing to electrode dislocation. The different approaches displayed in figure 49 were simulated in 2005 on the basis of a T1 weightened MRI scan of a patient at the Department of Stereotaxy and Functional Neurosurgery/ Cologne in collaboration with Prof. Sturm (Chairman of the Department). With the stereotactic planning software, a detailed analysis of the structures passed with the needle was possible (Figures 50 a-d). The accuracy of the planning is below the range of 1mm. The same computerized technique as clinically proven in deep brain electrode implantation in hundreds of patients with parkinsons disease was used.

3.   Results

3.1.   Retrospective ABI- study: data analysis

3.1.1.   Speech perception with auditory brainstem implants

Postoperatively 4 out of the 61 implanted patients did not receive useful auditory sensation when being stimulated. Two of these ("non-stim") patients received a contralateral ABI implant during tumor surgery over the following years and are now able to use this implant with benefit. No patient received any benefit from using both implants simultaneously. In contrast to other centers no non-stim patient was reoperated only with the purpose of improving the electrode position. After the initial "hookup" around 6 weeks after implantation, the patients variously described the sound from the ABI as muffled, like a towel over a loudspeaker, or like someone trying to talk with their mouth closed. Often, everything sounded the same at first. Even patients with high levels of speech recognition over years often showed relatively low levels of performance initially. Following a period of adaptation and learning, most patients reported a significant improvement in sound quality and performance.

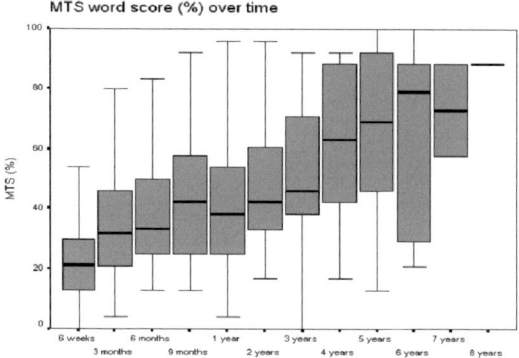

Figure 19: Box and Whisker plots showing the MTS test results over time, starting from the initial stimulation (approximately 6 weeks postoperatively) and continuing up to 8 years thereafter. Individual box-and-whisker plots show the 95th percentile range of scores and the mean scores (solid line). From: Otto SR, Kuchta J, et al, Journal of Neurosurgery, 2002.

Environmental sound recognition was at or above the 50% correct level in most patients (Figure 18). Patients typically found that the ability to discriminate and recognize environmental sounds was an early indication of benefit from their implants. Initially, patients are able to discriminate between environmental sounds on the basis of differing temporal patterns, such as the difference between a drum beat and a baby crying. With experience, some patients learn to discriminate beween sounds with similar temporal patterns on the basis of spectral information.

Several speech recognition tests were administered using sound from the ABI only. For word recognition (MTS-test), 87% of patients scored significantly above chance on closed-set word identification, and 98% scored significantly above chance on the recognition of the syllabe stress pattern (MTS-stress Test). These results demonstrate that ABI listeners were receiving amplitude, along with temporal and some spectral cues that facilitate spoken communication. However, most ABI users were unable to recognize words in sentences by using sound only. For most ABI patients the primary benefit in communication occurs when sound is used in conjunction with lipreading. The mean level of improvement over lipreading alone was 26% (range 0-66%). Thirty-one percent (17 of 55 patients) scored more than 70% correct in sound-plus-vision mode. Patients with more than 2 years of experience with an ABI generally perform better on all speech perception tests than those with less experience (Figure 19) . After several years of use, patients occasionally would begin to demonstrate some degree of open-set speech recognition.

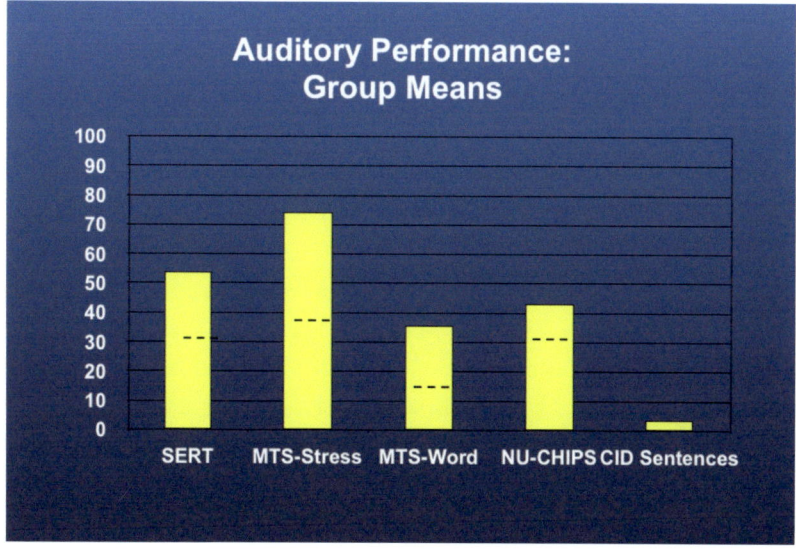

Figure 20: Perceptual performance results using the nucleus 24 ABI device (sound-only test condition without lip reading). Scores for SERT (sound effect recognition), MTS-Stress/ MTS-Word/NU-Chips (word recognition) and Sentence recognition scores for the sound-only condition are displayed. (n=58 patients).

3.1.2. Pitch range and perceptual performance

Pitch was not always easy for patients to discern, because electrodes rarely provided a pure tone like percept. It was usually the case, however, that patients could assign a pitch-related descriptor to the sounds (for example, bell-like, trumpet-like, bass drum-like). Pitch percepts on each electrode were assessed with magnitude scaling, in which a numeric scale from 1 to 100 units (low-to-high pitch) was used on a visual analogue scale. This was followed by eight pairwise pitch comparisons between electrodes. Pitch scaling provided a distribution of mean pitch scale values across electrodes and was able to reveal gaps in pitch ("holes in hearing") across the array. The SD of repeated pitch judgments could be used as an index of electrode distinctiveness. We found that gaps in pitch across electrodes could occasionally be filled by judicious selection of additional electrode pairs. Combinations of electrodes could sometimes produce a pitch intermediate to the individual ones of the component electrodes. Pitch scaling worked well as a precursor to pairwise comparisons between electrodes and provided a framework for the selection of electrode pairs for the task. Electrodes that did not sound identifiable different typically were not used and excluded from the stimulator map. This process usually resulted in a set of electrode channels that sounded identifiably different and were in proper pitch-rank order for use in configuring a sound processor map. Even though a big part of the primary tonotopic organization of the auditory brainstem extends below its surface, significant pitch information can be generated by surface stimulation. A predominant pattern of pitch distribution in ABI patients was a tendency for pitch to increase in a lateral-to-medial direction (electrodes 2-9) across the electrode array. This indicates some degree of consistency in the positioning of the ABI electrode array and in the structure of the cochlear nucleus relative to the electrode placement in the lateral recess. Nevertheless, we also found that a significant number of patients demonstrated a random or flattened pitch pattern as a function of electrode location.

GROUP	A	B	A	B	A	B
	N	N	Medium	Medium	Standard-deviation	Standard-deviation
CONS(S) %	25	29	20.48	21.62	14.37	13.96
VOWELS (S) %	25	29	29.80	31.83	16.23	17.10
CUNY SENTS (S) %	24	29	3.75	6.45	5.33	14.65
NUCHIPS	24	29	48.29	47.25	17.09	18.47
MTS WORD %	25	30	38.40	43.78	24.43	23.76

Table 1:Perceptual performance measurements (consonant, vowel, sentence and word recognition) in correlation to pitch range. Group A represents N=25 ABI patients who do not display significant pitch discrimination and/ or pitch range when beeing stimulated (Pitch range on a visual analogue scale between 0-100 was below 30). Group B represents N=30 ABI patients who demonstrated significant pitch discrimination and a pitch range of more than 30 on the visual analogue scale. Performance was significantly superior for group B patients only in the CUNY sentence recognition condition (6.45% versus 3.75%). The other conditions tested did not demonstrate any advantage of having a broad pitch range in N=55 ABI patients tested. (From Kuchta et al: 4th international conference on vestibular schwannomas, Cambridge, 2003).

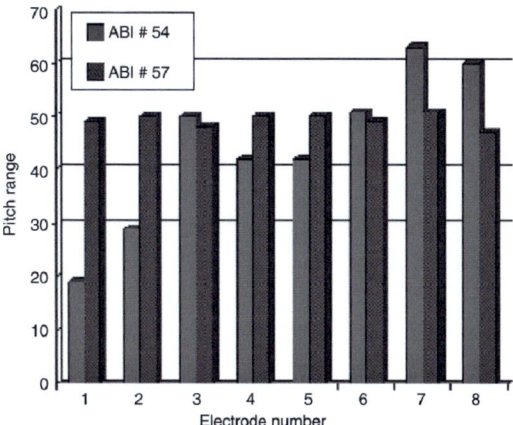

Figure 20:Pitch range in ABI patients. Exemplary patients (ABI#54, ABI#57) with flat (#57 and wide (#57) pitch range (Nucleus 8-channel ABI device).

A pitch range of more than 30 on the VAS was correlated with higher levels of sentence recognition. In word recognition as well as in consonant/vowel recognition no correlation between pitch range and perceptual performance was observed (see Table 1 above).

3.1.3. Side effects in auditory brainstem implantation

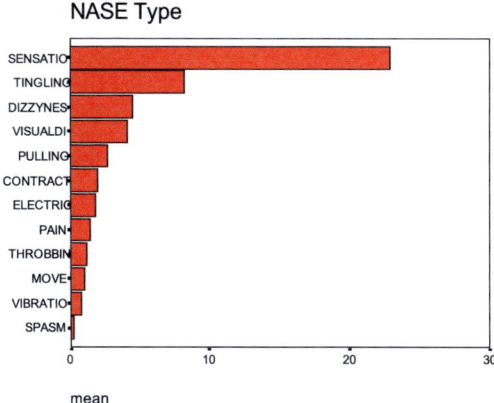

Figure 21:Sensoric and motoric non auditoriy side-effects (NASE) in N=440 audiological follow-up examinations. Nucleus 8-electrode ABI system, N=55 patients. The overall percentage of NASE is depicted on the X-axis. (Kuchta et al, Cambridge Conference on Vestibular schwannomas, 2003).

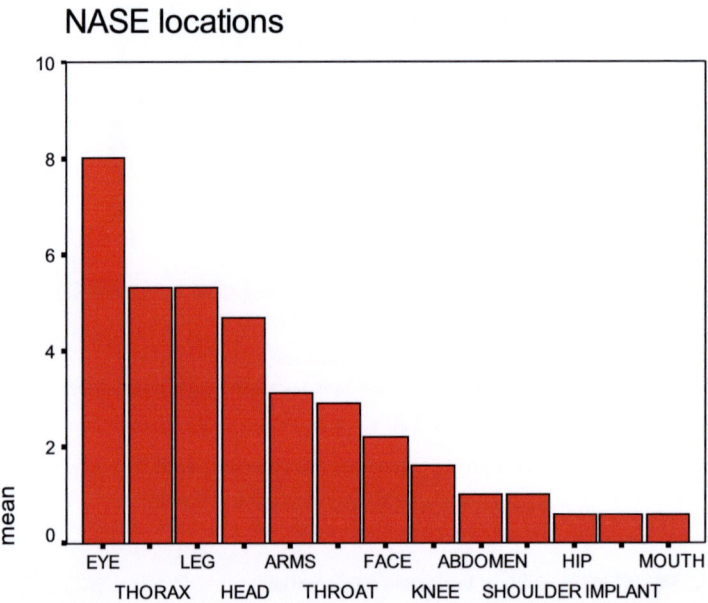

Figure 22: Locations of non auditory side-effects (NASE) in 440 audiological follow-up examinations. Nucleus 8-electrode ABI system, N=55 patients. The overall percentage of NASE is depicted on the Y-axis. (Kuchta et al, Cambridge Conference on vestibular schwannomas, 2003).

There were few significant complications in this series of 61 patients who underwent translabyrinthine microsurgery for ABI implantation and microneurosurgical removal of the vestibular schwannomas. As a complication of tumor removal, two of 61 patients experienced a cerebrospinal fluid leak that resolved after the application of a pressure dressing in one, and after lumbar drainage in the other. Infectious complications (meningitis) developed in one patient. We consider these to reflect general complications of cerebellopontine surgery. None of these complications were directly attributable to ABI implantation.

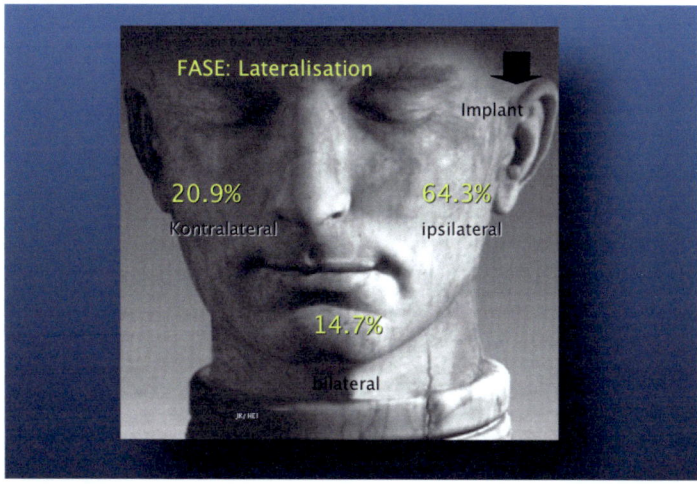

Figure 23: Lateralisation of Facial-nerve associated non-auditory side-effects (FASE/ activation of face muscles during ABI stimulation) in 6/119 ABI patients at the initial audiological testing and programming ("hook-up") around the 6th postoperative week.

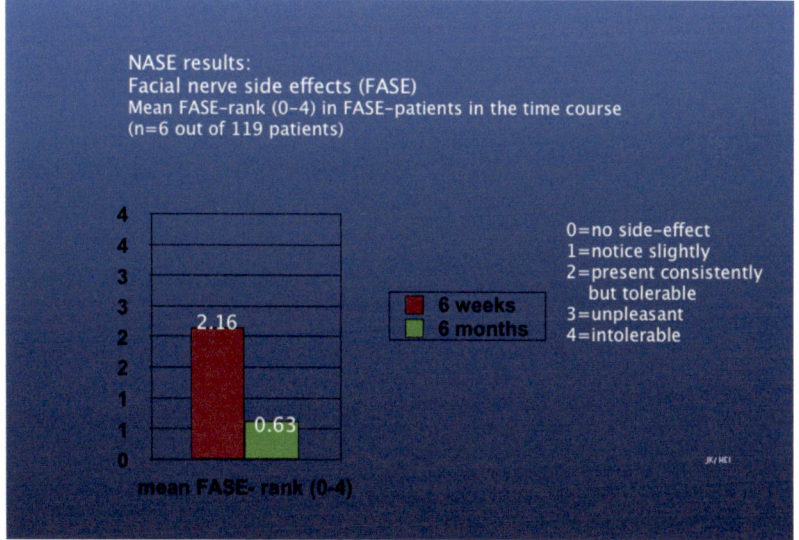

.Figure 24:Time course of Facial nerve side-effects (FASE) in 6/119 ABI patients. The columns represent the 6 week and 6 month time points. FASE decreased from 2.16 to 0.63 on average on the visual analogue scale (VAS 0-4)

Non-auditory side-effects (NASE) ranked 1-2 on the visual analogue scale were experienced in 68% of patients during the initial postoperative programming of the device. NASE were sensory in 93% and motoric in 7% of patients. Sensory NASE were mainly ipsilateral and included among others twitching or tingling sensations in the limbs and dizziness. Facial motor activity in reaction to stimulation of the device occurred in only 6.7% (6/119) of patients during the initial programming. Facial nerve side-effects decreased over time grade 2 (present consistently, but tolerable) 6 weeks postoperatively to grade 1 (notice slightly) on average at six months postoperatively (Figure 24). NASE were located ipsilateral to the side of implantation in most cases (Figure 23) and showed a tendency to be more pronounced at the lateral electrodes on the array. Minor nonauditory sensations detected at this stage (those ranked as "present consistently but tolerable") were reported but were generally not noticeable during actual sound processor use. More significant nonauditory sensations often could be managed by altering (usually increasing) the stimulus pulse duration, or by selecting a different ground electrode. If necessary, some electrodes could simply be deactivated to avoid nonauditory side effects completely. Nonauditory sensations decreased in magnitude over time in most patients.

3.1.4. The number of functional electrodes in auditory brainstem implants

*Number of auditory electrodes and perceptual performance**

Test	SERT	MTS SPR	Cons Recog	Vowels Recog	NU-CHIPS	MTS WR
chance level (%)	25	33	6	12.5	25	8
significantly above the level of chance (%)	41	53	9	26	38	19
mean test result (%)	55.8	75.7	20.4	28.8	51.8	41.1
range (%)	0–100	0–100	0–65	0–67	0–86	0–100
MNE (0–8)	1	1	2	3	1	3
MNEM (0–8)	1	1	3	3	3	3
MNEA (0–8)	2	3	5	5	6	8

* Cons = consonant; MNE = minimum number of auditory electrodes required for patients to perform significantly above the level of chance; MNEA = minimum number of electrodes in patients in whom performance becomes asymptotic; MNEM = minimum number of auditory electrodes needed for the mean performance of patients to be significantly above the level of chance; MTS SPR = MTS test, stress pattern recognition; MTS WR = MTS test, word recognition; NU-CHIPS = Northwestern University Children's Perception of Speech test (Elliott and Katz; 1980 [The task in this test is to identify the correct word from a set of four rhyming monosyllabic words presented in sound only.]); recog = recognition.

Table 2: The number of auditory electrodes and perceptual performance (from Kuchta et al, Journal of Neurosurgery, 2002).

Sound effect recognition test (SERT) scores: Recognition of environmental sounds like a doorbell or an approaching car is crucial in the daily life of secondary deafened patients. On the initial testing, discrimination and recognition of environmental sounds was an early indication of benefit from the implant and very motivating for patient and examiner since SERT performance was 60.82% on average (range: 27-100%, SD:15.83). Figure 25 shows the mean SERT scores of 61 auditory brainstem implant recipients. Postoperatively, 6 out of 61 implanted patients did not receive any auditory sensation when being stimulated ("non-stim.", number of auditory electrodes=0). But even with one functional auditory channel patients were able to discriminate environmental sounds significantly above chance (Figure 25). Most patients had more than 4 active electrodes. Range, standard deviation and variances were much higher in conditions with 5-8 electrodes. However, non-parametric tests and Mann-Whitney-U-Tests showed that the mean SERT performance did not significantly differ between the 1-8 electrode conditions ($p < 0.13$).

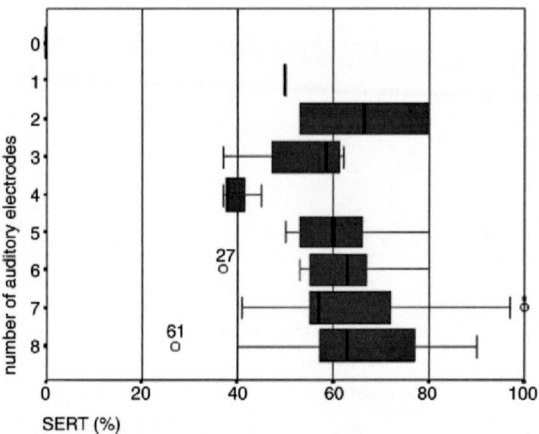

Figure 25: Sound effect recognition test (SERT) scores as a function of the number of active electrodes in 61 ABI patients. SERT requires the patient to choose from among five foils so that the chance performance level is at 20%. Single nonspeech sounds were not matched in their temporal patterns or frequency content, so that identification of their temporal pattern alone may allow correct identification. In this Box and Whisker plot the median is shown as the black line, the margins of the box represent the 25. and 75. percentile.

Consonants: To achieve sound-only sentence recognition, performance in the vowel and consonant tests has to approach 50% (Otto, personal communication). Figure 38a shows the mean consonant recognition scores of 61 auditory brainstem implant recipients. Mean performance increased as the number of electrodes increased from 4 (mean:8.0%, range: 4-11%, SD: 3.61) to 5 and above (mean: 21.67%, range: 4-65%, SD: 3.61). 2/3 of the patients with <3 spectral channels (electrodes) were able to perform significantly above chance level (13% and 23% resp.).

This finding seems consistent with previous work on consonant recognition in the complete absence of spectral cues (Rosen et al., 1992; Shannon et al., 1995; Turner et al., 1995; van Tassel et al., 1992) demonstrating that significant consonant identification can be achieved with only temporal cues. Nevertheless, higher (>20%) scores on consonant recognition seem to be possible only with more than 4 electrodes. High variability was observed in the scores with 5-8 electrodes. Differences between the 1-8 electrode conditions did not reach statistical significance in non-parametric tests and Mann-Whitney-U-Tests (P>0.12).

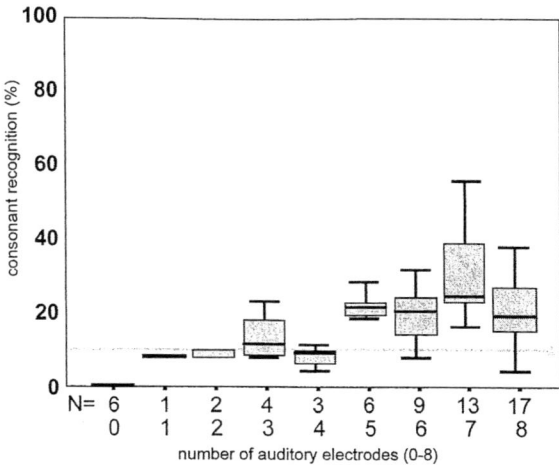

Figure 26a: Recognition of 14 medial consonants in a (a/C/a) context as a function of the number of electrodes for 61 nucleus 22 patients. Mean scores (black line), 25/75 percentiles (box) and number of patients for every condition are shown (N=1-17).

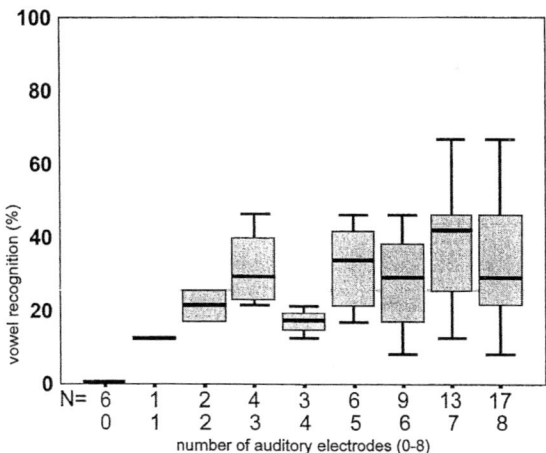

Figure 26b: Recognition of 8 vowels in a (h/V/d) context as a function of the number of electrodes in 61 nucleus-22 patients. Mean scores (black line), 25/75 percentiles (box) and number of patients for every condition are shown.

Vowels: Recognition of vowels is shown in Figure 26b. Mean vowel identification of all conditions was 28.31% (range:0-67%, SD:16.17). The level of vowel identification for the 1-electrode condition was lower (12%, n=1) than for the 2-4 electrode condition (mean: 21.42%, range: 4-33%, n=9), but on non-parametric tests and Mann-Whitney-U Tests these differences were not statistically significant (p=0.157). Similar to the consonant recognition test, however, the ten top-performers had more than 4 usable electrodes. No further increase was observed with electrode numbers above 7; mean performance in patients with eight electrodes (33.53%, N=17, range: 8-67%, SD: 18.66) was even 3.78% below the 7-electrode condition (37.31%, n=13, range: 12-67%, SD: 18.08).

From cochlear implant studies (Fishman et al., 1998) it is known that implant listeners tend to use more spectral information in vowel recognition than in consonant recognition. There are relatively fewer differences in duration and amplitude among vowels than among consonants. Consonants recognition by implant users may be more dependent on temporal cues than vowel recognition and so may be identifiable with relatively few spectral information, i.e. fewer electrodes. MTS- word recognition was scored for both word recognition and for stress patterns correct (Figure 27 a+b). In the MTS word recognition task (Figure 27a) the mean score for all conditions was 44.78% (range:13-100%, SD:22.96). The patients with only one or two electrodes were not able to perform significantly above chance in the word recognition task (mean: 15%, range 13-17%), but were able to recognize on average 74.67% of constituent stress patterns (range: 72-89%, Figure 39b). Word recognition increased by 22.75% when the patients had 3 or more auditory electrodes available. For the 6-8- electrode condition, mean listener performance was 50.33% correct with a range from 13% to 100%. Mean MTS stress-pattern recognition score (Figure 27b) was 82.58% (range: 50-100%, SD: 23.66) and increased only slightly from mean 71% correct with 1 electrode to 77% (range: 29-96%) with 4 electrodes. Word recognition improved only little as the number of available channels increased to 8 (mean: 82,58%, range: 50-100%). There was no statistically significant difference between performance with 1-8 electrode in stress pattern recognition (P>0.15). In contrast to MTS word recognition, vowel and sentence recognition tests, top-performance for MTS stress pattern recognition could also be achieved with only 3 available electrodes/ spectral channels.

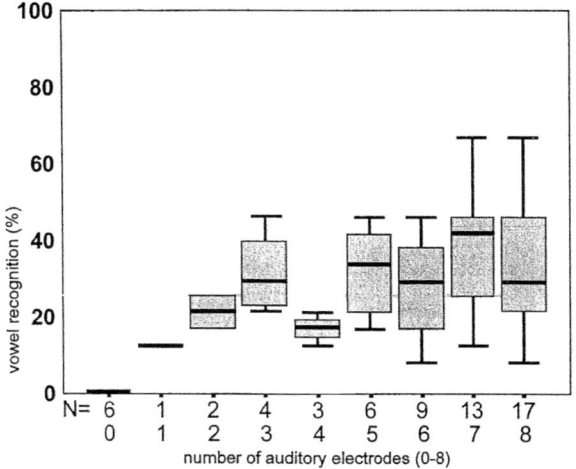

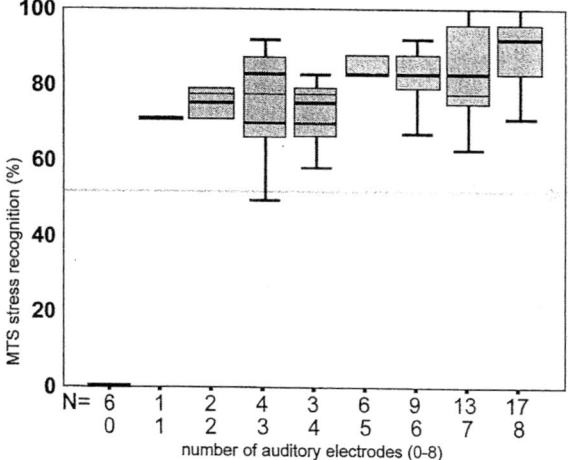

Figure 27 a+b: MTS-word and MTS-stress recognition: The Monosyllable, Spondee, Trochee (MTS) test consists of 12 words that differ in the number of syllables (monosyllable vs. others) and in the stress patterns in two-syllable words (spondee vs. trochee). The patients results are evaluated both in terms of stress patterns correct (Figure 27b) and number of words correct (Figure 27a). Mean scores (black line), 25/75 percentiles (box) and number of patients for every condition are shown.

CUNY Sentences (Figure 28): Mean perceptual performance with 8-channel ABI patients was (only!) 1.07% (range:0-64%, SD: 11.44). Performance was virtually zero with 0-3 electrodes (n: 13, range: 0-2%, SD:12.92%) and increased to 2.67% on average (range:0-7%, SD:.3.79) with 4 auditory electrodes. Perceptual performance in sentence recognition increased further up to 10% on average with all 8 electrodes available. Like in most other test conditions the top performers had 6-8 functional auditory electrodes providing spectral information.

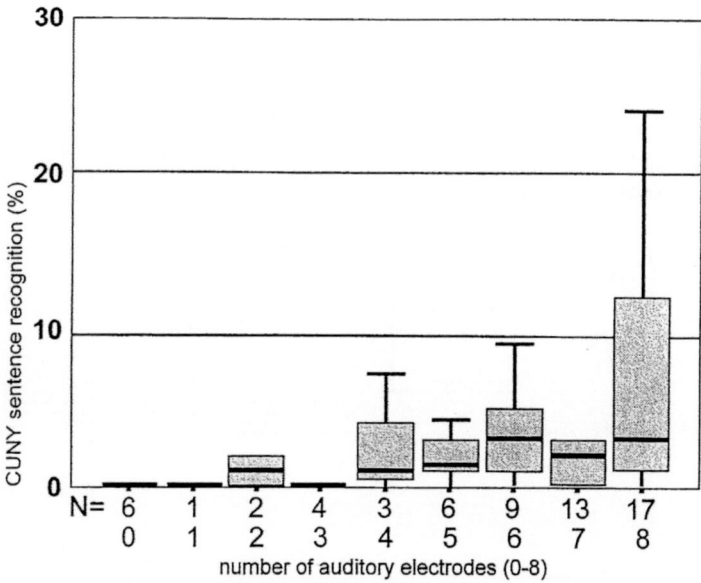

Figure 28: CUNY results for sentence recognition: CUNY (City University of New York Sentences, Tyler/Preece et al 1987) tests results in the sound-only condition. Mean scores (black line), 25/75 percentiles (box) and number of patients for every condition are shown.

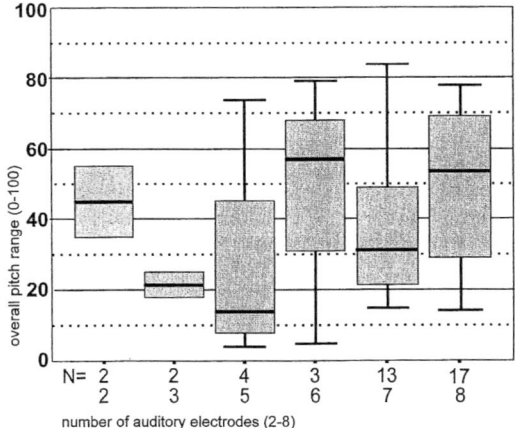

Figure 29:Overall pitch range as a function of the number of electrodes. During the initial fitting of the device pitch sensations on specific electrodes were assessed on a visual analog scale ranging 1-100 and electrodes were ranked in the order of the evoked pitch sensation. Overall pitch range was defined as the range (0-100) from the lowest to the highest pitch on the visual analog scale. Mean scores (black line), 25/75 percentiles (box) and number of patients for every condition are shown.

Since in patients with only one active auditory channel no pitch range can be assessed, only the results with two or more auditory electrodes are displayed in Figure 29. Differences in pitch range between electrode numbers were not statistically significant (p<0.39). Even with only two functional auditory electrodes on the array, patients are able to perceive significant pitch differences (35 and 55/100 respective). However, in 3/12 of the 8-electrode patients and 3/11 of the 7-electrode patients no clear pitch difference (range=<20/100) between the electrodes was found. After the individual pitch ranking is performed, the auditory electrodes are ordered according to their relative frequency. In some patients we (J.K.+ S.O.) examined the importance of this pitch ranking for the individual performance. Re-arranging the order of the available electrodes in the "wrong" order caused a significant decrease of speech perception. Perceptual performance with only two auditory electrodes arranged in the adequate order was better than performance with 8 functional electrodes which were not assigned to the adequate spectral band. The main part of this "electrode number" study was performed with NF2 patients who received the 8-channel device, which is the device most commonly used between 1990 and 2000. We (J.K.+ S.O.) also had the chance to review the perceptual performance data of the first 9 patients who received the newer 21-channel electrode device. Speech recognition was also tested in the SERT, MTS, Consonant, Vowel and CUNY sentence recognition task. Surprisingly no significant advantage could be detected for the 21-channel model when compared to the older 8-channel model. Increasing the number of possible spectral channels from 8 to 21 did not result in higher levels of performance (Figure 30).

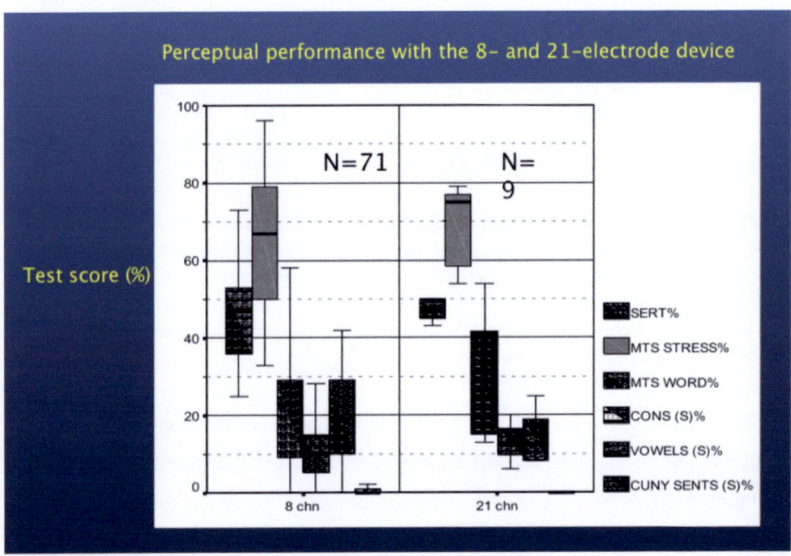

Figure 30: Comparison of the 8- and the 21-electrode ABI concerning perceptual performance measurements (SERT, MTS, consonants, vowels and sentence recognition). No significant improvement in performance was achieved by increasing the number of functional electrodes from 8 to 21. Speech recognition scores of 71 8-channel ABI patients and 8 21-electrode ABI patients are displayed.

3.1.5 Auditory brainstem implants after previous radiosurgery

6 of the ABI implanted patients had a history of previous gamma knife surgery on the implanted side. One patient had a history of previous proton beam radiation.

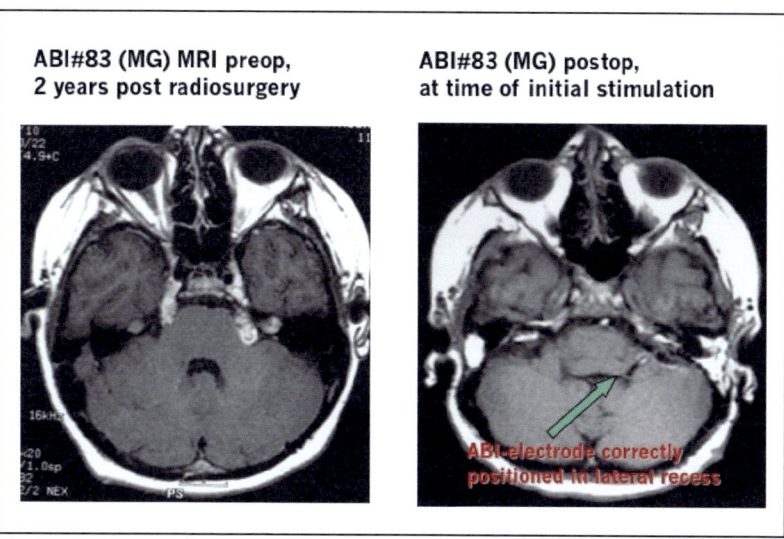

Figure 31: Preoperative and postoperative MRI-scan of a patient with a vestibular schwannoma in the left CPA. The left image shows tumor progression in spite of performed convergent beam irradiation (CBI) 2 years after radiosurgery. On the right side the postoperative status after resection of the VS and microsurgical ABI implantation into the lateral recess is displayed. The patient was able to discriminate environmental sounds and showed a significantly improved lip reading score when using the ABI. Consonant and word recognition scores were above average (Figure 32).

Three out of six preoperatively irradiated patients from HEI were able to use their device every day with benefit. However, these cases are to be evaluated carefully preoperatively with auditory evoked potentials (AEP) and intraoperatively with electrical evoked auditory brainstem responses (EABR) to determine the potential viability of the structures in the cochlear nucleus region.

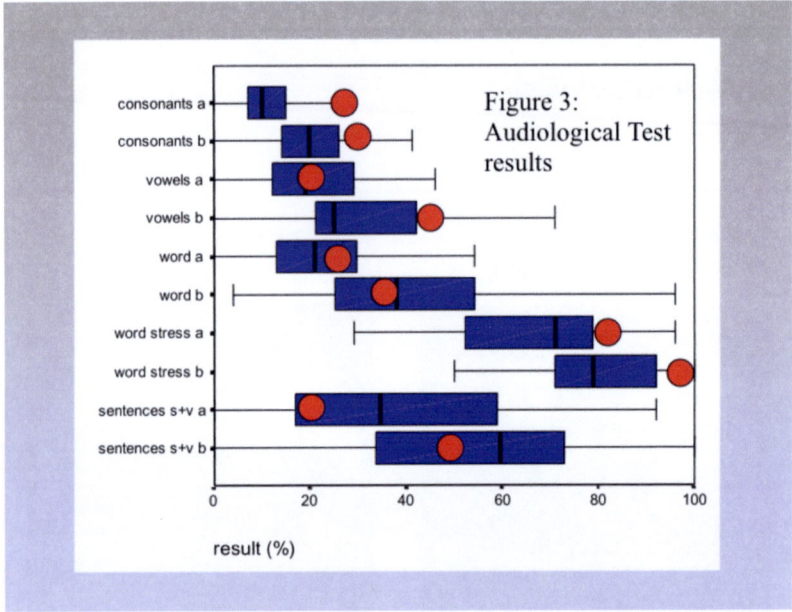

Figure 32:Box and whisker plot summarizing the postoperative audiological results of 119 patients that were implanted with an auditory brainstem implant at HEI. Consonant recognition, vowel recognition, MTS-word recognition scores were all tested "sound only". CUNY-sentence recognition was tested "sound only" and "sound+vision". Results of two different follow-up examinations are displayed: A= initial stimulation at 6 weeks postoperative, B= 6 months follow-up testing., The circles represent the perceptual performance results of the post Gamma-knife patient "MG" (ABI #83). This post radiosurgery patient also showed the typical effects of learning and reprogramming with significantly improved scores in the follow up after 6 months (from Kuchta et al, American Associaton of Neurosurgeons (AANS) meeting, San Diego, 2001).

3.1.6. International comparison of ABI outcome

In Europe, the retrosigmoid approach is used much more frequently for ABI implantation when compared to the the translabyrinthine (TL) approach. All patients who received auditory percepts demonstrated improved speech recognition in combination with lip reading. A limited number of patients achieved some open-set sound-only speech recognition. The European patients showed better scores in the visual-only condition, i.e. they were better lip readers (37.3%/ 22.5%). Overall perceptual performance measurements were better in the european group although the heterogenity of the audiological tests performed makes direct comparison of the test results impractible.

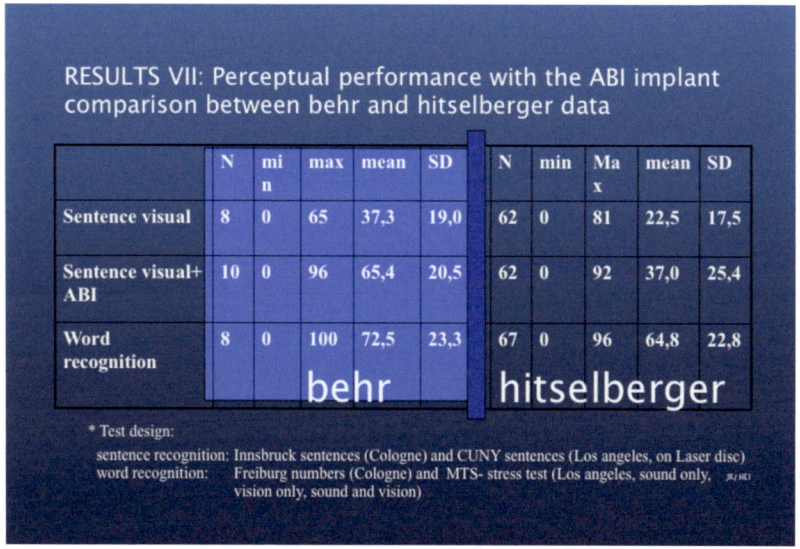

	N	min	max	mean	SD		N	min	Max	mean	SD
Sentence visual	8	0	65	37,3	19,0		62	0	81	22,5	17,5
Sentence visual+ ABI	10	0	96	65,4	20,5		62	0	92	37,0	25,4
Word recognition	8	0	100	72,5	23,3		67	0	96	64,8	22,8

RESULTS VII: Perceptual performance with the ABI implant comparison between behr and hitselberger data

behr   hitselberger

* Test design:
sentence recognition: Innsbruck sentences (Cologne) and CUNY sentences (Los angeles, on Laser disc)
word recognition: Freiburg numbers (Cologne) and MTS- stress test (Los angeles, sound only,
                     vision only, sound and vision)

Figure 33: Here the perceptual performance scores of N=10 exemplary European patients using the Med-el ABI system (implanting surgeon: Robert Behr) and N=67 American patients using the Nucleus system (implanting surgeon: William Hitselberger, personal communication, Chapter 3.1.1) were compared. Word recognition scores in the sound only condition were 72.5% on average in the "Behr" group and 64.8% in the "Hitselberger" group.

Test scores for sentence recognition in the visual and ABI combined mode came out much better in the European patients than in the American patients. The "Behr" patients turned out to be better lip-readers (sentence recognition in the visual only mode). Mean scores for sentence recognition with lip reading were 37.5% in the "Behr" group and 22.5% in the Los Angeles group. Non-auditory side effects under stimulation as described and analyzed in chapter 2.1.1 were not observed in the "Behr" patients. No complains about tingling, dizzyness, visual disturbance, pulling, muscle contraction, electric sensations, pain, vibration or spasm were reported. The reason for this may be differences in electrode placement or programming of the device.

3.2.   Imaging study

3.2.1. Postoperative electrode position

Postoperative imaging with MRI and/or CT was obtained in 58 out of 119 patients. The ABI device was full compatible with magnetic fields up to 1.5 Tesla without any direct or delayed ABI-related side-effects being reported by the patients. The MRI-artefact resulting from the ABI electrode and implanted receiver/stimulator device has become significantly reduced since the magnet was removed from the Nucleus-24 receiver coil at the time of surgery. Patients now use a small tape retainer disk that contains a thin piece of metal placed on a shaved area of the scalp directly over the receiver/stimulator antenna. This technique allows high-resolution MRI studies to monitor the postoperative status of multiple tumors in NF2 patients. We (J.K., W.L., J.F.) were able to assess and document the position of the implanted ABI array in relation to anatomic landmarks in 46 out of the 58 postoperative image studies.

Electrodes were placed over the ventral cochlear nucleus in 14%, over the dorsal cochlear nucleus in 16%, deep in the recessus in the direction of the 4th ventricle in 30% and at the entrance of the lateral recessus in 40% (Figure 34). With all electrode positions there were patients performing significantly above chance. The best auditory performance was correlated with electrode placement close to the ventral cochlear nucleus over the taenia choroidei (column 1 in Figure 34). With deep placement, non-auditory side-effects like dizziness were more common, probably due to collateral stimulation of the inferior cerebellar peduncle and the vestibular nuclei. Since no magnets were used for coil fixation, magnetic resonance imaging (MRI) can be performed to follow tumor progression. In the first years CT was used to evaluate the position of the ABI electrode in relation to bony landmarks and to assess the long-term stability of the ABI electrode.

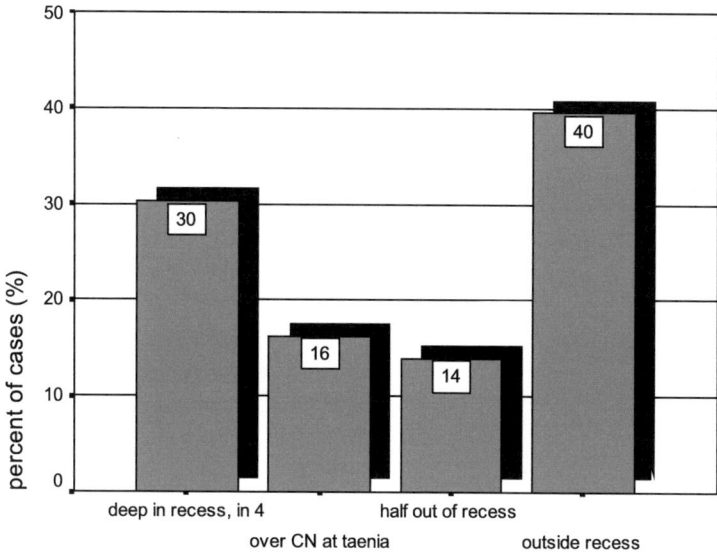

Figure 34: Postoperative electrode positions in 46 ABI patients based on the postoperative imaging (MRI/CT). Most electrode postions were classified as suboptimal ("deep in the recess" or "outside recess". Only around one third of electrodes were positioned optimal ("over CN at taenia" or "half out of recess") according to the targeted region during implantation.

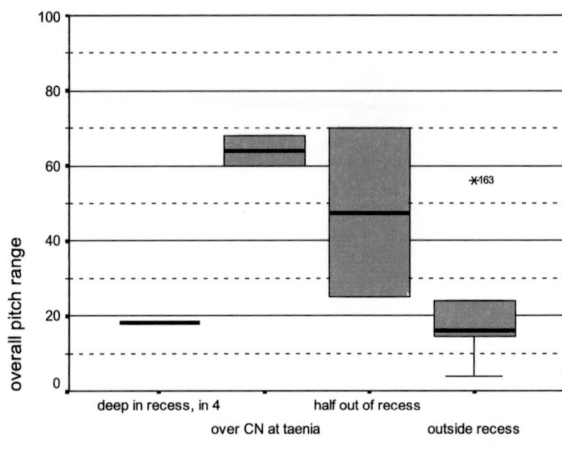

Figure 35: Overall pitch range in correlation to electrode postion (N=46 ABI patients). Pitch range was optimal in the "over CN at taenia" and "half out of recess" positions.

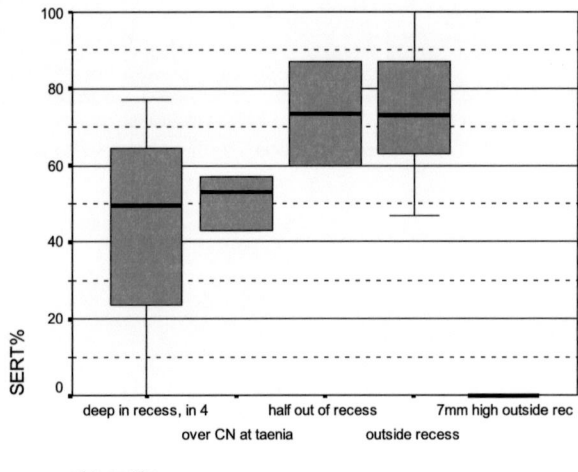

Figure 36: Sound effect recognition test results (SERT) in correlation to postoperative electrode positions. The best SERT results were obtained in the "half out of recess" and "outside recess" positions (N=46 ABI patients).

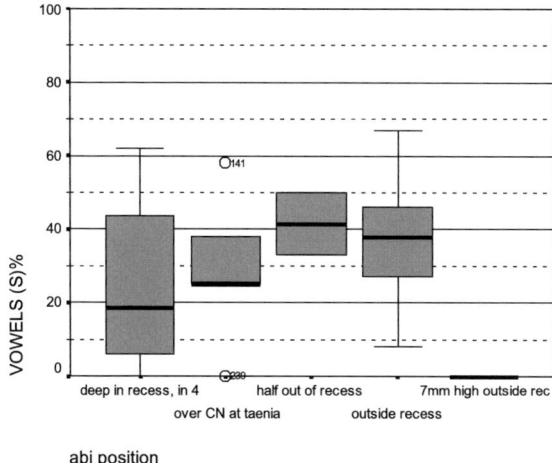

Figure 37: Vowel recognition scores in corellation to postoperative electrode positions. The best vowel recognition scores were obtained in the "half out of recess" position (N=46 ABI patients) recognition scores were obtained in the "half out of recess" position (N=46 ABI patients).

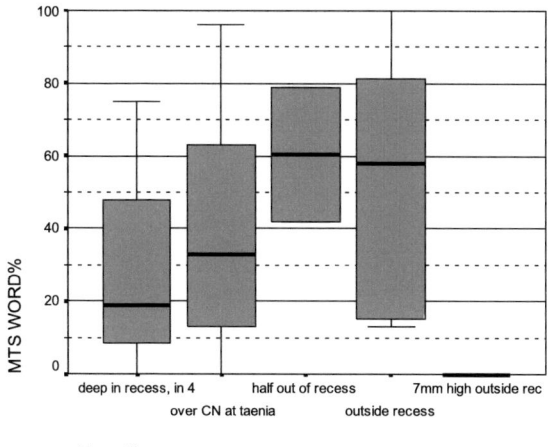

Figure 38: MTS word recognition scores in corellation to postoperative electrode positions (N=46 ABI patients)

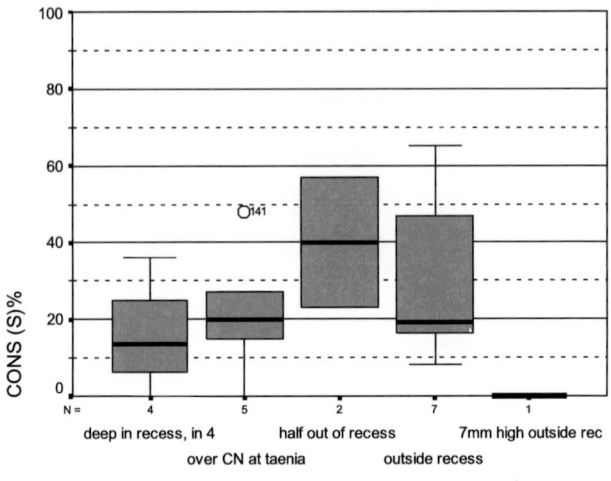

Figure 39: Consonant recognition scores in correlation to postoperative electrode positions. The best recognition scores were obtained in the „half out of recess" position (N=46 ABI patients).

Concerning the overall postoperative position (Figure 34), most electrodes were classified as suboptimal ("deep in the recess" or "outside recess"). Only around one third of electrodes were positioned optimal according to the targeted region intraoperatively ("over CN at taenia" or "half out of recess"). This may reflect the tendency of the surgeon to achieve a secure position of the implanted electrode inside the lateral recess. Positions deep inside the recess may be more stable and show less electrode migration in the postoperative follow-up. Concerning the overall pitch range (Figure 35), there was a huge, statistically significant difference among the different electrode positions. ABI patients with electrode positions deep inside the lateral recess of the 4th ventricle do not achieve an overall pitch range above 20 (on the VAS from 0-100). Positions "over CN at taenia" and "half out of recess" were correlated to much higher pitch ranges. These patients have more spectral information available, which seems to be a precondition for higher levels of speech recognition. This advantage in spectral information must be put in relation to the disadvantageous mechanical characteristics and more difficult fixation of the electrode at a position "half out of the recess". Concerning the sound effect recognition scores (SERT, Figure 36), vowel (Figure 37) and MTS- word (Figure

38) scores, the best results were obtained with postions "half out the recess". This electrode position is in close relationship to the ventral part of the cochlear nucleus. Based on this postoperative imaging study in relation to the postoperative perceptual results, the ventral cochlear nuclueus seems to be the structure providing the highest levels of speech recognition. The VCN seems to be the ideal target for neuroprosthetic stimulation with the auditory brainstem implant. Having the possibility of an electrode dislocation in mind (see next chapter), the surgeon has to make a compromise between mechanical stability (optimal with deep implantation inside the lateral recess) and perceptual performance (optimal with electrode positions directly at the entrance of the lateral recess) in each individual patient.

3.2.2. Stability of the electrode-brain interface

The number of electrodes providing auditory sensation remained very stable in most ABI recipients when it was re-evaluated after 3-36 months. In 44/61 patients there was no change in the number of functional electrodes on the array in the time course. In 7 patients the electrode number increased by one and in 6 patients it decreased by one electrode in the time course. In 4 out of 61 patients, the number of functional electrodes increased by more than 1. No patient "lost" more than 1 electrode in the time course. These changes of electrode number were not statistically significant.

3.2.3. The impact on lateral recess anatomy on perceptual performance

The lateral recess as assedded intraoperatively by the implanting surgeon (W.H.) was „small" in 17/65, "medium" in 25/65, "large" in 19/65 and "huge" in 4/65 patients. Unsatisfactory performance was significantly correlated to "large" and "huge" size of the lateral recess. Patients with large or huge lateral recessus show sub-average perceptual ABI performance (Table 3, Figure 40). This fact may be due to reduced functional integrity of the central auditory pathways, unfavourable impedance of the electrode/ tissue contact surface, or postoperative movement of the electrodes.

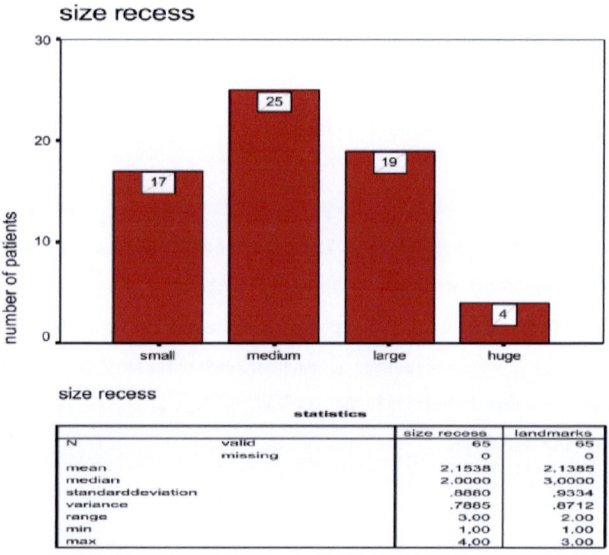

Figure 40: The size of the lateral recess in N=65 ABI patient (distribution) based on the intraoperative estimation by the surgeon (WH).

Deskriptive Statistik

size recess		N	Minimum	Maximum	Mittelwert	Standardab weichung
small	CONS (S)%	10	5	20	11,10	5,00
	VOWELS (S)%	10	12	33	19,70	8,67
	MTS WORD%	10	8	54	22,50	13,32
	CIDSENTS	9	0	2	,22	,67
	Gültige Werte (Listenweise)	9				
medium	CONS (S)%	14	0	31	13,50	8,22
	VOWELS (S)%	14	8	42	21,86	11,11
	MTS WORD%	15	4	71	26,73	20,42
	CIDSENTS	13	0	2	,15	,55
	Gültige Werte (Listenweise)	13				
large	CONS (S)%	11	0	28	9,00	7,63
	VOWELS (S)%	11	0	42	17,82	11,51
	MTS WORD%	11	0	29	18,45	10,42
	CIDSENTS	9	0	0	,00	,00
	Gültige Werte (Listenweise)	9				
huge	CONS (S)%	1	0	0	,00	.
	VOWELS (S)%	1	0	0	,00	,
	MTS WORD%	2	0	46	23,00	32,53
	CIDSENTS	0				
	Gültige Werte (Listenweise)	0				

Table 3: Perceptual performance measurements (consonant, vowel, word and sentence recognition scores) in relation to relative size of the lateral recess. N=65 ABI patients.

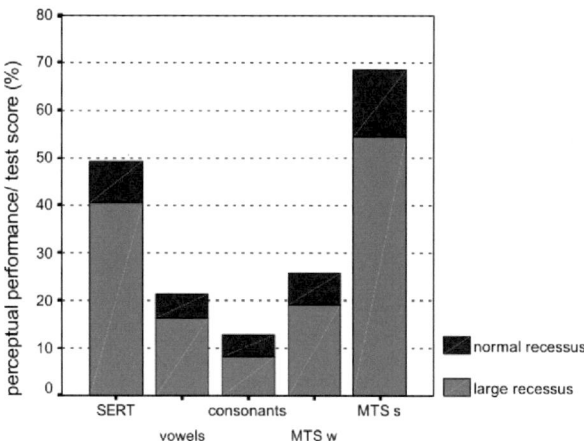

Figure 41: Perceptual performance measurements (consonant, vowel, word and sentence recognition scores) in relation to the relative size of the lateral recess. N=65 ABI patients.

ABI- Electrode positions with normal and large lateral recessus

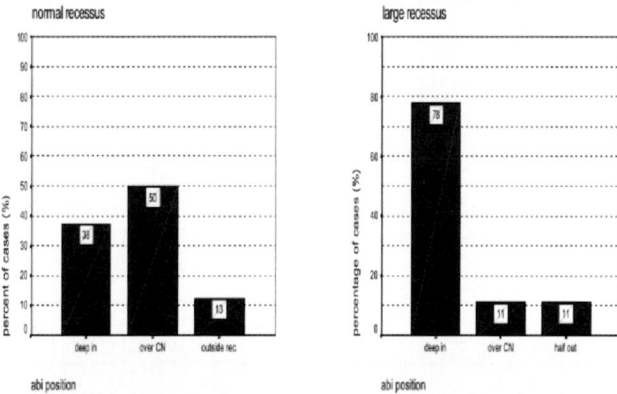

Figure 42: Postoperative electrode positons in relation to the relative size of the lateral recess (N=65 ABI patients).

Figure 42 shows that in about 4/5 of cases with a large lateral recess, the final electrode position based on the postoperative imaging (see previous chapter) was deep inside the lateral recess.

3.3.   Electrophysiological study

3.3.1. Intraoperative Neural response telemetry (NRT)

For a classification of the NRT responses please see chapter 2.3.1. and 4.3.2. In 25.7% a questionable response (class 3-5) and in 25.7% no NRT responses (class 0-2) were recorded with monopolar stimulation. Using the bipolar protocol (Figure 44b) only in 11.8% clear responses (class 6-8), in 35.3% a questionable (class 3-5) and in 55.9% no responses (class 0-2) were obtained. While stimulating the same locations with EABR in 75% clear responses, in 13.9% questionable response and in 11.1% no responses were obtained. The recorded CAP response was very small when compared to the current used for stimulation.

Therefore the response passes through an amplifier which is switched on automatically after the stimulus artefact has decayed. We (J.K. and S.O.) have found that the measurement delay which can be specified is very critical for the clarity of the NRT response. To avoid amplifier saturation due to the stimulus artefact, the delay should be long enough until the stimulus artefact has decayed sufficiently. With a long delay, on the other hand, early components of the CAP (such as the N1 peak) which latencies are typically around 200-300 us after the stimulus (probe) onset may disappear. After testing various delays in the range of 35-80 us in implanted volunteers, we found that a delay of 50 us seems most appropriate since it shows all the early components of the NRT response without distorting the trace due to amplifier saturation. In contrast to cochlear implant NRT results, no clear class-8 responses (biological, including N1) were found in our 7 patients tested intraoperatively. NRT waveforms were very heterogenous among individual patients and also among different electrodes. These cross-electrode differences may reflect the differences in the temporal response capabilities of the stimulated neural populations. A typical intra-operative NRT response was correlated to a typical intra-operative EABR response in 75% of cases.

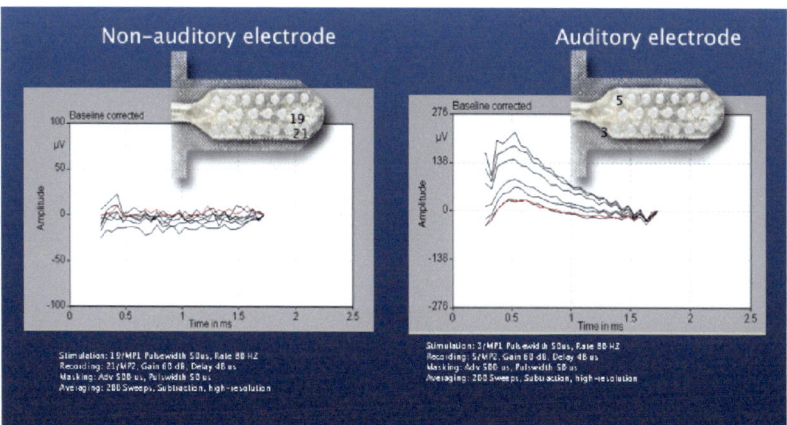

Figure 43: Exemplary NRT recordings from ABI patient #108. Comparison of compound action potential responses as a result from stimulating on one electrode on the array and recording from a neighbouring electrode. This technique was applied intraoperatively as well as postoperatively for the first time in ABI patients to provide an electric "mapping" of the electrode carrier (J.K. and SO). No clear responses were obtained from a region that postoperatively provided no auditory percepts (left). Clear "cochlear-like" responses were obtained from regions that later turned out to provide auditory sensations (right). Stimulation parameters: Pulsewidth 50 μs, Rate 80 Hz, Gain 60 dB. Recording parameters: Gain 6 dB, Delay 48 μs, Masking parameters: Adv 500 μs, Pulswith 50 μs. Averaging parameters: 200 Sweeps, Subtraction mode, high resolution.

Five of the patients on which intraoperative measurements were performed have been re-tested at the initial hookup session at 6 weeks postoperatively. In 4 out of 5 patients the NRT responses remained unchanged (clear CI-like responses, class 6-8, please see response classification in chapter 4.3.2., Table 5). Only in one patient the responses type changed slightly from class 6 (biological response, low amplitude) to 5 (ski-slope pattern, questionable response).

With acoustic click stimuli unit latencies in the VIII nerve and all ABR wave latencies decrease with stimulus intensity as much as 2 ms when the stimulus amplitude varies between threshold and saturation. In our NRT recordings we have not seen this inverse correlation between stimulus amplitude and the latency of the response. In cochlear implants the electrically evoked compound action potential frequently show a double peak waveform. Stypulkowski et al (1984) suggested that the double peak complex may be due to two underlying individual response components (axonal and dendritic). In our intraoperative NRT recordings only single peak CAP responses were observed.

Intraoperative Neural Response Telemetry
Monopolar protocol

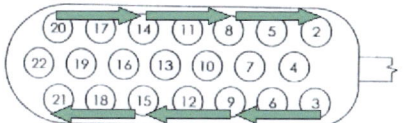

Stim/Rec Parameters:

20-14	21-15
14-8	15-9
8-2	9-3

Stimulation: MP1 Reference,
Pulsewidth 50us, Rate 80 HZ
Recording: MP2 Reference,
Gain 60 dB, Delay 50 us
Masking: Advance 500 us,
Pulswidth 50 us
Averaging: 200 Sweeps, Subtraction,
High resolution

Intraoperative Neural Response Telemetry
Bipolar protocol   Stim/Rec Parameters:

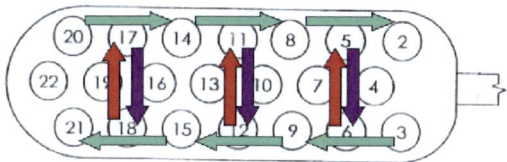

Stim:	2,8	8,14	14,20	21,15	15,9	9,3
Rec:	6,mp1	12,mp1	18,mp1	17,mp1	11,mp1	5,mp1

Figure 44a+ b: Monopolar and bipolar intraoperative mapping protocol used for the recording of compound action potentials in ABI patients (developed by Kuchta/ Waring 2001). Using these protocols, a complete "map" of the electrode carrier was obtained in each patient, representing the neural response telemetric pattern ot the individual electrodes.

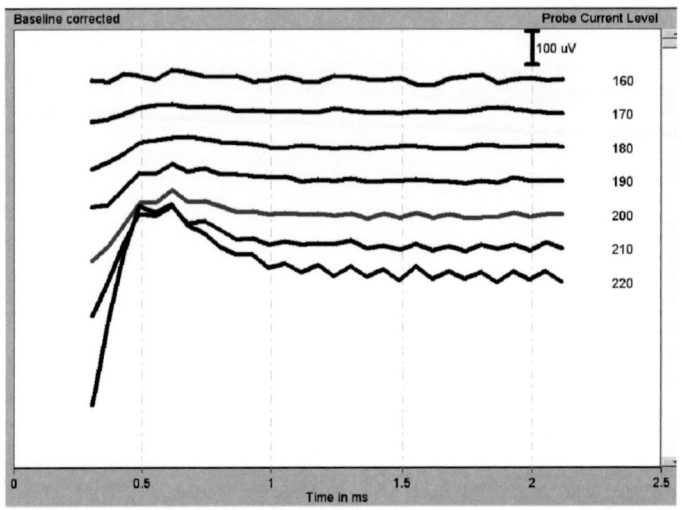

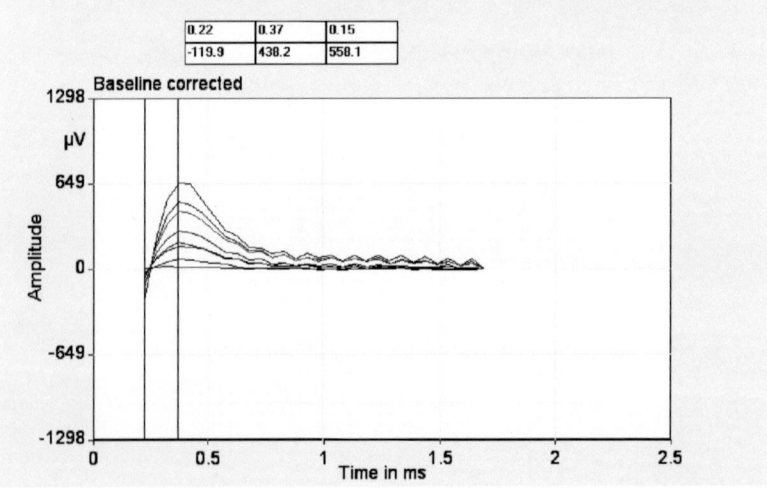

Figure 45a+b: CRP Waveforms: Electrically evoked whole nerve action potential growth functions obtained using the neural response telemetry system of the Nucleus CI24M device (Cochlear Corporation). The panel shows a series of waveforms, the responses have been offset from each other. The parameter on this figure is the stimulation current level in device programming units. In the amplitude growth function displayed below, the increasing amplitude of the NRT response is shown with increasing stimulus amplitude (from Kuchta et al: Biomedizinische Technik, 2004).

At the postoperative testing and programming session, the impedance of the stimulation and recording site are measured on a regular basis. Impedances can be calculated using the WinDPS software and should be neither excessive (hig impedance) or too low (short cut). We (J.K. and S.O.) suggest to exclude NRT measurements with high impedance (>20 kΩ, shown as "open" by the WinDPS) from the analysis. Intraoperatively, automatic monitoring of the impedance at the recording sites is not implemented in NRT v2.04 but will be in a later software release according to Cochlear corporation.

The complete NRT mapping of the electrode carrier took 12 minutes and 45 seconds on average (4.50-21.20 minutes). After the first test runs measurements were faster due to training and acommodation to the NRT system in the environment of the operation room. The measurement of a complete amplitude growth function took about 50 seconds for every electrode combination. Clear NRT responses were obtained in all 7 patients and in 46.8 % of all regions tested (6 per electrode carrier, stimulation pattern according to Fig 44). The latency of the NRT peaks varied between 0,28 and 0,60 ms (mean= 0,456 ms, SD= 0,1218). The amplitudes of the NRT responses varied between 140 and 1250 mV (mean=359 mV, SD=245,78) (Figure 45). All 5 patients tested postoperatively had clear biological (class 6-7, see chapter 4.3.2.) NRT responses on at least one electrode (6 measurements per patients, monopolar protocol Figure 12, overall 30 postop NRT recordings). Post-operative NRT thresholds were always at levels audible to patients. Electrode misplacement may be detected due to the occurrence of unusual patterns of the compound action potential. Our comparison of intraoperative and postoperative waveforms showed a high intraindividual stability. There were some correlations between the intraoperative NRT thresholds and the postoperative psychophysical thresholds (T- and C-level).

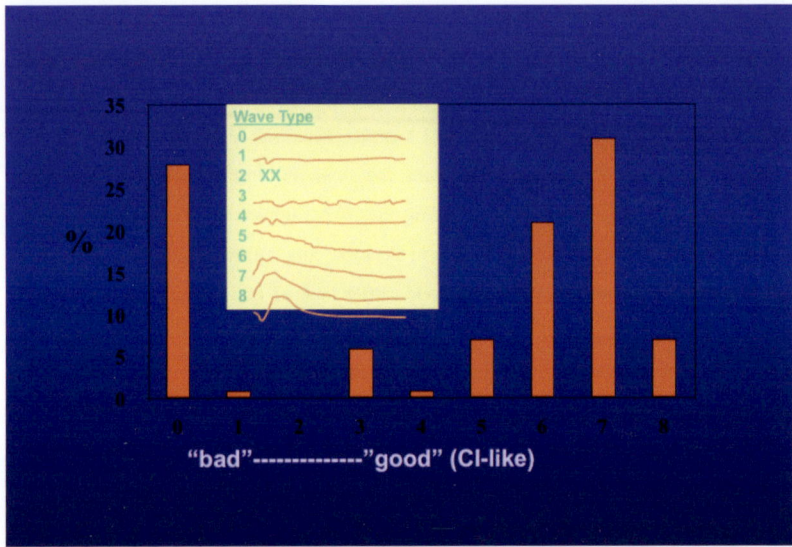

Figure 46: Description and distribution of NRT Responses class 0-8, see also NRT- response classification, page 36. (N=99 postoperative NRT recordings in 17 AB-patients, 21-channel Nucleus ABI).

3.4.   Laboratory studies:

3.4.1. Implantation and MRI- imaging of a prototype PABI electrode in human cadaver heads

The translabyrinthine approach provides a good angle of exposure and enables penetrating electrode positioning using the applicator developed at the HMRI. The TL requires minimal cerebellar retraction and allows early identification of the facial nerve during the operation. Postoperatively the electrodes could be localized in the lateral recess using the imaging technique described above. Both, the surface and the penetrating ABI electrodes were compatible with MRI imaging. In the fututre more elaborated MRI sequences may be used to further reduce the metal artifact produced by both implants. Due to resulting artefact from the metal and air inclusions, the two electrodes could not be differentiated very well (Figure 47).

Image fusion techniques (Chapter 1.4.3., Department of Stereotaxy and Functional Neurosurgery) providing a combination of MRI and CT may possibly further improve postoperative electrode localization and preoperative planning.

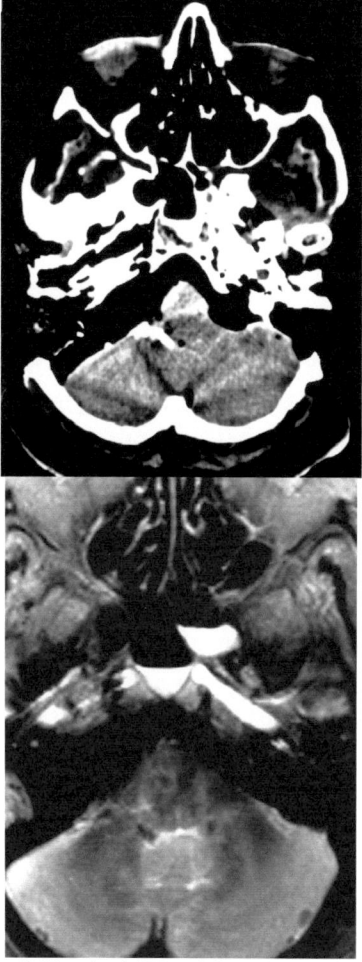

Figure 47: Axial CCT scan (left) and axial T2-weightened scan of a cadaver head specimen. A penetrating ABI electrode (PABI) was implanted in combination with a surface ABI electrode inside the lateral recess of the 4th ventricle via a translabyrinthine approach using the applicator tool developed at HMRI (Figure 12).

3.4.2. Animal studies: Implantation and stimulation of the IC

Cortical multi- unit activity was recorded in response to electrical stimulation at the IC. The experiment was started by recording neural activity in the IC in response to acoustic stimulation. Cortical positions with the best recordings in response to acoustic stimulation were used also for stimulation at the IC. Biphasic charge-balanced pulses between 1-200uA (mean: 100uA) were then used for stimulation of the IC laminae with the HMRI microelectrodes described in chapter 2.4.1.. Cortical multi- unit activity was recorded in response to electrical stimulation at the level of the IC. Individual spikes as well as an averaged negative deflection was detected. The duration of the electrically evoked cortical responses was between 10 and 30ms. Spike activity increased parallel to increasing stimulus levels at the IC. Stimulation thresholds for stimulation at the IC were between 30 and 70 uA, which results in a total charge density per phase below 10nC. The overall charge density per phase at the stimulation site was between 1 and 10uC/cm. Activity of small clusters of neurons or single neurons was amplified, band-pass filtered, and monitored on an oscilloscope. Spike activity was isolated from the background noise with a window discriminator. A detailed cortical threshold mapping was not performed in this study due to the limited time for reliable recordings in this acute study. Negative deflections from the baseline were defined as the recorded responses. The latency was taken as the time between the stimulus and the negative peak. The electrical threshold for stimulation was defined as the current level of stimulation at the IC that elicts visually distinguishable cortical spikes. Cortical potentials were averaged across 100 trials on each cortical recording site. The area of successful recordings was limited to the region between the anterior and posterior sylvian sulcus, in the rostrocaudal direction, and between the supra-sylvian sulcus and the dorsal tips of the anterior sylvian sulcus. In general, regions that showed low response thresholds and continued physiologically viable status of the cat brain´s surface were used.

3.4.3. Engineering: Developement of a prototype stereotactic auditory deep brain electrode

The results of the electrode number study (chapter 3.1.4.) were very important for the design of the SAI. Although speech recognition in ABI is possible with only 4 spectral channels, a stimulating stereotactic auditory implant should have 8-12 electrodes incorporated to provide sufficient frequency selective auditory information to the IC. Similar to ABI surface stimulation, not all electrodes will be functional and provide auditory sensations. The engineering task was to arrange the 12 electrodes on a thin needle-type electrode carrier. The advantages of ring-electrodes as well as plate electrodes were discussed in our interdisciplinary team (J.K., C.J., S.N.) at Med-El. Two prototype needle-type electrodes with 12 individual contacts were manufactured. The total diameter of the SAI electrode is 1.25 mm. On both sides of the carrier, 6 plate electrode were fixed. The lenght of the complete array carrying the electrodes is 5mm (Figure 47-48).

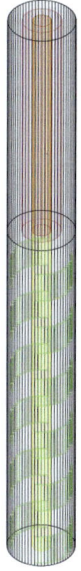

Figure 48a: Design of a ABI electrode for minimally invasive application into the central auditory pathways (Type A, circular shape with 12 plate electrodes).

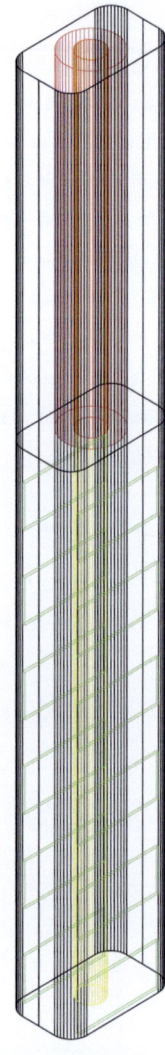

Figure 48b: Design of an ABI electrode for minimally invasive application into the central auditory pathways (Type B, non-circular shape with 12 plate electrodes).

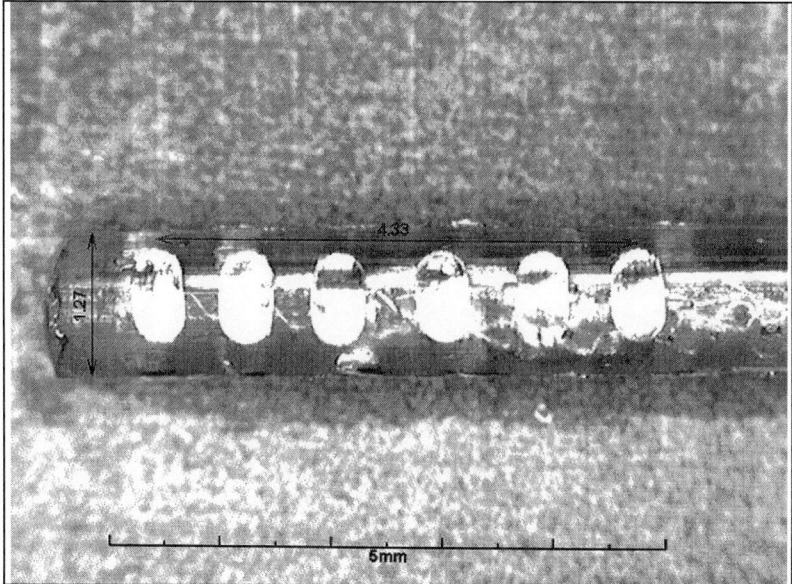

Figure 49: Microscopic photograph of the SAI electrode tip (Johannes Kuchta, Cologne University/ Claude Jolly, MedEl). The prototype #685 has an 0.20 mm Nitinol wire as stylet, which is super-flexible but not very rigid. A second prototype (#699) has an 0.25 mm steel wire as stylet, which is much more rigid than the Nitinol but not as flexible.

The actual electrode tip has 12 channels (6 on each side), 1.1 mm channel spacing. The electrode is virtually round in cross section and is tapered. Since the electrode tip has to penetrate through the brain tissue when inserted beyond the end of the guide tube, we prefer the more stiff electrode (#699, Figure 49 above). We were aiming to two rows of stimulation contacts with each contact being designated to its own channel (i.e. frequency band). Initially also a partially flat electrode that does not twist easily during or after implantation was designed (Figure 48b). The diameter of this electrode was 1.3x 0.8 mm. For electrode dimensions as mentioned above, the range of stimulation per channel would be about 0.2 mm.

3.4.4. MRI- based stereotactic approach for IC implantation

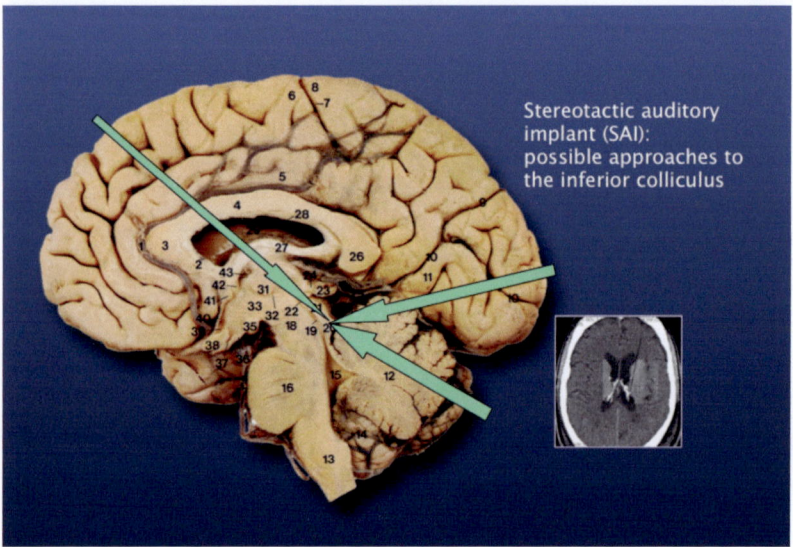

Figure 50: Possible stereotactic approaches to the inferior colliculus (SAI-project): A: dorsal infratentorial transcerebellar approach (DITA), B: dorsal suboccipital transtentorial approach (DSTA), C: frontal transcerebral approach (FTCA).

The clinical application of the first stereotactic ABI implant (SAI) is planned after the prototype electrode has been connected to the commerically available Med-El ABI system and approval of the Ethic´s committee of Cologne University has been obtained. The operation can be carried out with local anaesthesia. The semi-flexible electrode (diameter 1.2 mm) will be implanted into the inferior colliculus using stereotactic planning software (chapter 1.4.3.) through a frontal burr-hole on the right. The external receiver/stimulator device will be implanted subcutaneously under the clavicle similar to a cardiac pacemaker. Audiologic tests and reprogramming of the device will be performed six weeks postoperatively and after 6, 12 and 24 months. The pre- and postoperative audiological testing will be performed by Martin Walger and Johannes Kuchta in collaboration with Robert Shannon and Steve Otto/ House Ear Institute. Concerning the stereotactic approach to the inferior colliculus, the first intention was to use the dorsal infratentorial transcerebellar approach (DITA, Figure 50) because this seemed to be the anatomically shortest way to the midbrain. This approach has also been used in our group in the laboratory studies in the cat as described in chapter 2.4.2.. The DITA approach is a widely used neurosurgical approach for the resection of lesions in the pineal region. Concerning the stereotactic implantation of deep brain electrodes, this approach has several disadvantages. The first problem concerns the positioning of the patient. The dorsal transcerebellar approach would require a positioning "upside down" or in the "park bench" position to perform the burr hole trephination and the placement of the electrode. This is very cumbersome for the patient as well as for the surgeon. It is probably impossible to carry out a deep brain implantation via the DITA approach in local anaesthesia, which is required for having the best level of intraoperative monitoring and patient feetback.

The second problem concerns the stability of the implanted electrode: Using the DITA approach, the electrode will pass the CSF filled cisterna before penetrating the midbrain. These different characteristics of the changing media on the way to the IC (brain- CSF- brain) are probably disadvantageous concerning the fixation of the electrode. The SAI electrode implanted via the DITA approach may be more sensible to movement and dislocation. Because of these disadvantages of the dorsal approaches, we now favour a frontal transcortical approach (FTCA) for SAI implantation. Placement of the deep brain electrode while the patient is positioned comfortably in the supine position promised to be very relaxing for the patient as well as for the surgeon.

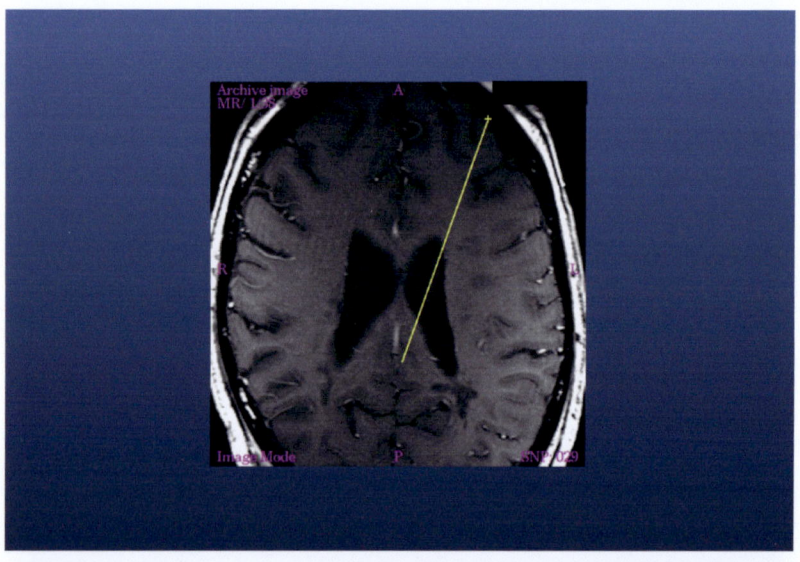

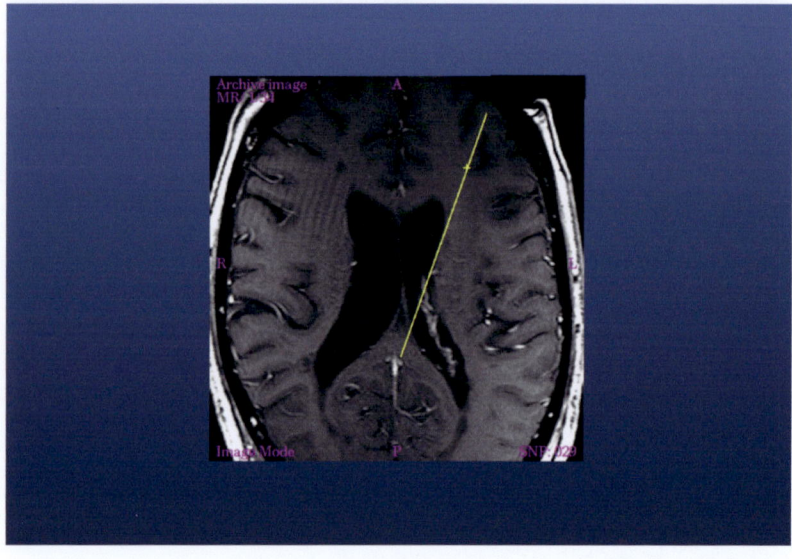

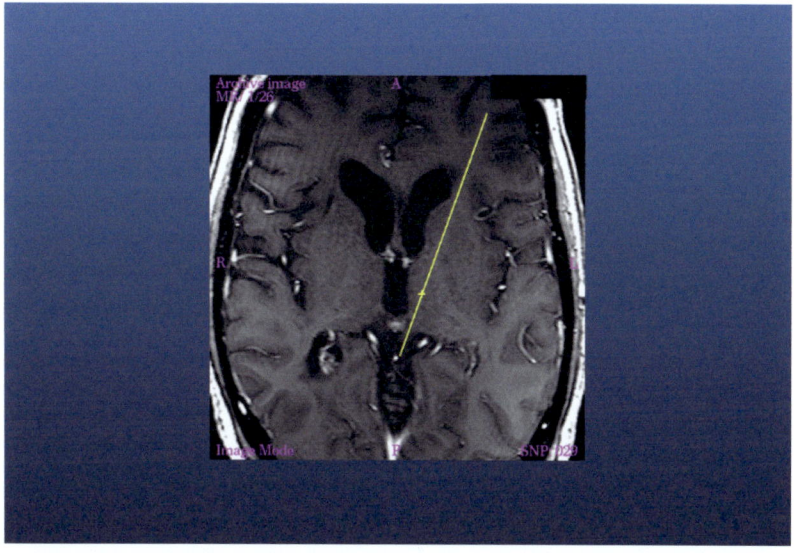

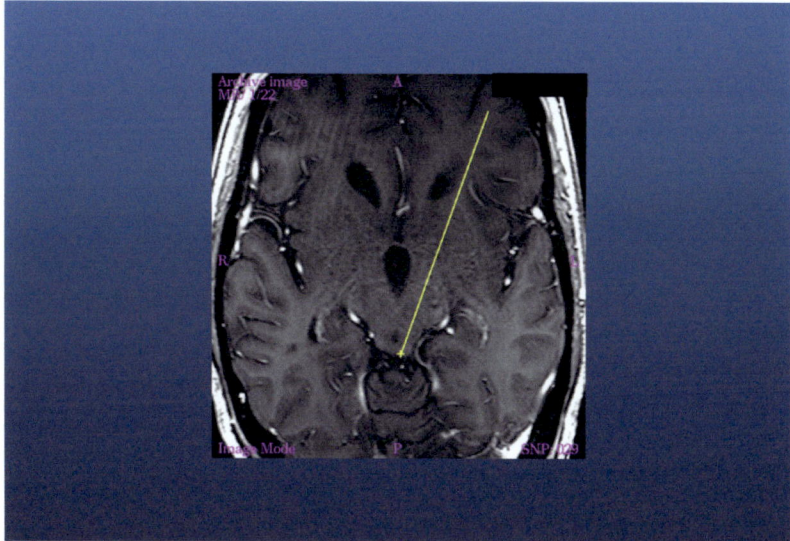

Figure 51 a-d: Trajectory of the planned stereotactic approach (frontal transcerebral approach) on the basis of axial T1- weightened MRI scans. (Johannes Kuchta/ Volker Sturm, 2005).

4.   Discussion

4.1.   Discussion of ABI performance study results

The degree of environmental sound discrimination and speech recognition is very variable among ABI recipients. While several patients obtain a relatively high level of sound-only speech perception, the majority perform at lower levels. Even more than in cochlear implantation, the perceptual performance of these patients is dependent on a variety of individual factors such as the survival of neurons in the cochlear nuclei, differences in surgical placement, anatomic variations, experience, and the ability to capitalize on modest auditory cues.

The structures stimulated by an electrode in the brainstem may depend on several anatomical and physiological factors that each influence the auditory outcome. Earlier reported studies (Terr et al, 1989, McCreery et al, 1997) have shown that the ABI electrode is fixed in the lateral recess by fibrous tissue during the first postoperative days. This encapsulating tissue may significantly add resistance to the spread of current from the array to the stimulated neurons and may be a reason for elevated thresholds or missing auditory sensation in some cases. Another critical factor is the number of viable, stimulable neurons in the cochlear nucleus after years of deafness. A clear relation between the duration of preoperative deafness and post-implant perceptual performance was not observed, so that even long-lasting preoperative deafness is not considered to be a contraindication for central auditory implantation. Non-auditory sensations are generated by the spread of current to non-auditory structures in the brainstem. Since the range of stimulation from the tip of the electrode is about 1mm/mA, assuming the maximal applicable current of 2mA with the ABI possible sites of stimulation have to be located within approximately 2mm (Figure 8).

Concerning the facial nerve, direct stimulation with the result of ipsilateral motoric activation of the facial muscles is possible. Nevertheless, this is very unlikely since the facial nerve is more than 2mm away from the cochlear nucleus and from the ABI electrodes located in the lateral recess of the fourth ventricle. Direct facial nerve stimulation is therefore only possible when the electrode carrier has been significantly displaced, or has migrated from its initial position. One of the closest structures in relation to the implanted electrode carrier that is not crossed at this point in the brainstem (most FASE are ipsilateral to the stimulating electrode(!)) is the inferior peduncle of the cerebellum.

Since the inferior cerebellar peduncle is an ascending fibre tract, stimulation above threshold can evoke tingling sensations in the extremities in some patients. By antidromic activation of the inferior cerebellar peduncle the action potentials may also travel distally and cause motor side-effects in the extremities or in the facial region. The occurrence of non- auditory side-effects (NASE), and especially facial nerve associated side-effects (FASE), does complicate the postoperative fitting of the device and requires a time-consuming individual testing and programming of the sound processor. Testing and programming will require many hours of concentration and interaction with the patient. Intensive and frank preoperative consulting of the patients is especially important in ABI implantation to avoid unreasonably high expectations and to establish a trustful relation between the patient, the patient´s family and all the medical personal involved. Facial nerve associated side-effects (FASE) in auditory brainstem implants are a surprisingly rare finding. FASE can be managed by changing the pulsewidth or by switching off the electrode channels from the map in most cases. Since the remaining FASE (rank 3-4) show a tendency to decrease over time in almost all (98.3%) cases they do not represent a serious complication of brainstem stimulation. Intraoperative monitoring with EMG, electrical evoked far-field potentials (EABR) and maybe NRT (chapter 2.3.1) may further reduce the occurrence of non-auditory side effects by assisting electrode placement and assessing the stimulability of the auditory neurons. Due to technical advances and increasing experience in interpreting the obtained intra-operative responses, intra-operative monitoring with electrically evoked auditory brainstem responses (EABR) has become a helpful tool in assisting the surgeon, especially in cases with difficult anatomy and long-lasting deafness. With preserved intra-operative EABR (evoked from the electrode array or a removable probe electrode), the likelihood of getting significant postoperative benefit from the ABI device is very high even in patients with a history of previous radiosurgery.

In cochlear implants group data across all tests showed significant improvements in speech recognition as the number of electrodes was increased from 1 to 4 electrodes (Fishmann et al., 1998). Patients implanted with the electrode array implanted close to the surface of the cochlear nucleus showed a similar pattern when tested for vowel, MTS word, and CUNY sentence recognition. However when tested for Sound effect recognition, consonants and

MTS stress pattern recognition this correlation of perceptual performance and the number of available electrodes was not observed.

In these tests patients were able to perform above chance level with only one functional auditory electrode. This is probably due to the fact that performance above chance is possible with only temporal cues in these tests. The top-ten performers, however, were always in the group with a higher number of functional auditory electrodes.

The importance of the number of electrodes has been investigated by several different researchers (Lawson et al., 1996; Dorman et al., 1989). Lawson et al found a significant improvement of consonant recognition as the number of electrodes was increased from 1 to 4, but no clear difference between the 4-22 electrode conditions. Fishman et al. (1997) created processors with different numbers of electrodes by assigning the outputs of multiple analysis filters to a single electrode. For example, a 4-electrode processor was created by routing the outputs of filters 1-5 to electrode 3, filters 6-10 to electrode 8, filters 11-15 to electrode 13, and filters 16-20 to electrode 18. They reported that performance on a variety of speech recognition tasks improved as the number of electrodes increased from 1 up to 7, but then no change in performance was observed as the number of electrodes was increased from 7 to 20. They argued that, although spectral information was available from 20 frequency bands, implant listeners were not utilizing all of the potential spectral cues presented on the 20 electrodes. Similar findings on the effect of the number of electrodes have been observed with other implant devices, such as Ineraid (Dorman et al., 1989; Lawson et al., 1993), Med-El Combi 40 (Brill et al., 1997), Nucleus-22 with a percutaneous connector (Lawson et al., Reference Note 3), Nucleus-22 with the f0/f1/f2 speech processing strategy (Holmes et al., 1987; Kileny et al., 1992), and with normal-hearing listeners who were restricted in the number of spectral channels (Dorman et al., 1997b; Hill et al., 1968; Shannon et al., 1995). These previous studies demonstrated that multi-channel cochlear implants provide better speech recognition than single-channel cochlear implants, primarily because subjects with multi-channel devices receive spectral or place cues in speech signals in addition to the temporal cues provided by single channel devices (Fishman et al., 1997). In cochlear implant patients it has been shown that patients with more electrode interaction contain lower speech recognition scores (Hanekom and Shannon, 1996). In general, electrical current spread should be greater at higher stimulation levels and for monopolar stimulation modes. However, other studies (Kileny et al.,1992; Zwolan et al, 1996) have shown that the same or even better speech perception can be obtained with monopolar stimulation modes.

Increasing the number of electrodes above a critical number on the small carrier array may also increase the amount of electrode interaction that limits ABI performance, thereby resulting in an asymptotic or even deteriorating performance above a certain electrode number. Although a certain amount of spectral information is provided by the independently stimulated electrodes, the cochlear nucleus may only be able to utilize spectral information up to a "critical mass". The fact that speech recognition in ABI users seems not to be strictly correlated to the number of auditory electrodes on the array in the 2-4 electrode conditions is in contrast to cochlear implant stimulation, where a   statistically significant difference between these conditions was found in all tests. ABI performance is in general poorer than cochlear implant performance, probably because the surface electrodes of the present ABI are only incompletely capable of stimulating the tonotopic axis of the cochlear nucleus. The problem mentioned above is the primary motivating factor for the development and future clinical application of penetrating microelectrodes for the cochlear nucleus (PABI, chapter 1.3.) or the inferior colliculus (IC, chapter 2.4.1.). PABI can stimulate highly selective areas of the human cochlear nucleus, obtain better access to the tonotopic lamina of the cochlear nucleus and thereby may overcome this major shortcoming of systems stimulating only the surface of the cochlear nucleus.

ABI recipients seem to have only a limited capability to utilize the spectral information provided by the ABI multi-electrode surface array when compared with cochlear implantation. In speech recognition tests that require spectral cues to perform above chance (vowel, MTS word and CUNY sentence recognition), a minimum of three functional auditory electrodes providing spectral information seem to be necessary for satisfactory performance. When the surface of the cochlear nucleus was stimulated with more than 6 spectral channels (functional electrodes), performance levels showed an asymptotic behaviour in most tests. We assume that the reason for this asymptotic characteristic is the limited access to the tonotopic axis of the ventral cochlear nucleus being the target area for stimulation. Other factors like electrode interactions on the contact surface of the array seem less likely. Experiments in which the number of auditory electrodes was varied in a controlled manner showed a significant correlation of perceptual performance and electrode number. Even more crucial for speech perception than the mere number of electrodes is the appropriate ranking of spectral bands to the individual electrodes.

Penetrating electrodes for the cochlear nucleus and the inferior colliculus will probably overcome some of these limitations associated with surface electrodes and may further improve ABI performance by   providing a wider tonotopic range and improved specificity. When comparing the Los Angeles results with the European ("Behr") group- the "Behr" patients turned out to be better lip-readers (sentence recognition in the visual only mode). Mean scores for sentence recognition with lip reading were 37.5% in the European group and 22.5% in the Los Angeles group. A reliable comparison of score in differend countries is very difficult because totally different performance scores were used, each varying in the level of chance performance. In the United States most tests were performed in a standardized fashion using a computer program or a video disc of the same speaker. In most European trials, the test were performed "life" by the individual audiologist, which may bring some variable and subjective bias to test performance.

4.2. Discussion of imaging study results

The possibility that a shift in position of the brainstem after removal of the tumor mass would cause a change in the electrode position relative to the targeted brainstem structures has been an issue of concern. Over time, a fibrous connective tissue capsule forms around the electrode array. A fibrotic capsule was observed surrounding and infiltrating an electrode array that was removed from one of the early patients 22 months after implantation (Terr et al, 1989). Histologic examination of the capsule indicated that it was fibroblastic in nature and highly invasive of the Dacron mesh carrier. It is not known how much time is required for such a capsule to form in patients; heavy connective tissue ingrowth of Dacron mesh carriers occurs in experimental animals within 2 weeks of implantation. However, once the brain has shifted to its normal position and the electrodes are encapsulated in fibrous tissue, further movement of the device is very unlikely.Radiologic evidence from follow-up CT and MRI scans attest to a high degree of positional stability of the electrode array. Probably the close fit of the electrode array into the lateral recess holds the electrode assembly in position during the critical days immediately after implantation, while fibrous tissue is invading the Dacron carrier and fixing the electrode in place. Electrode migration or dislocation does not represent a problem in the follow up period between 6 weeks (initial hookup) and the following 8 years in the patients examined here. No clear information can be assessed about electrode migration in the first postoperative days since no neuroradiologic imaging and no audiologic tests were performed during this time. According to the results from chapter 3.2.1, this is not an ideal position to achieve high levels of perceptual performance. In concordance to the situation described in chapter 2.9.2, the surgeon has to choose between putting the electrode very deep in the lateral recessus (which is probably the more stable position), or position the ABI at the entrace of the lateral ventricle (which is more instable, but correlated to better speech recognition). This dilemma becomes even more important in patients with large or huge lateral recess (chapter 3.2.1). According to the results in chapter 2.2.1, a preoperative measurement of the lateral recess based on preoperative MRI scans make sense, because this condition is associated with sub-average speech recognition levels. Regarding the fixation of the electrode in the lateral recess, the technique of Dr. Hitselberger and Prof. Behr is different. In L.A., the ABI electrode carrier is kept in place by pushing it half-way into the recess and covering it with a layer of teflon, which brings some positional stability. In addition to this, Prof. Behr uses fibrin glue to fix the electrode carrier after the functionality has been tested with intraoperative neuromonitoring (EABR). This may add stability to the electrode- nerve interface and may prevent postoperative dislocation of the implant. According to results in chapter 3.1.1, pre-implant radiosurgery is not necessary correlated with bad audiological outcome after auditory brainstem implantation. If modern stereotactic planning and treatment techniques are used and the radiation damage is restricted to the acoustic nerve, the outcome is similar to that in non-radiated patients. With severe brainstem damage as seen with pre-computer aided radiation plans or proton beam radiation, the patients do not benefit very much from the implant. Recently some good results were also achieved in some patients who underwent previous radiosurgery for their vestibular schwannomas, a condition previously considered a contraindication to ABI implantation. Although the audiological results are below average and the operation may be more difficult than in non-irradiated patients, preoperative radiosurgery should not be considered as a contraindication to ABI implantation in all cases.

4.3. Discussion of electrophysiological results

Between different individuals using the ABI,   there is a wide range of performance (chapter 3.1.1.). Duration of deafness, cognitive processing strategies, properties of the residual auditory system and the age of the patient are factors influencing audiological outcome. The most critical factors are probably nerve survival and electrode placement. Intraoperative functional electrophysiologic monitoring of the stimulated pathways is an important tool for the surgeon. We have shown in chapter 3.3.1. for the first time, that it is possible to record individual CAP waveforms and CAP growth functions from the ABI electrode carrier both intraoperatively and postoperatively. In all patients where the ABI was able to provide auditory sensations a clear NRT response was recorded from the electrode carrier. 44% of the post-operative NRT records obtained in this study were not "CI-like" in morphology, showing either "no response" or "questionable response". Nevertheless, almost half of these non-"CI-like" waveforms were associated with stimulation that elicited hearing sensations. This would create a dilemma regarding whether to reposition the ABI electrode array intra-operatively if the NRT waveform showed no clear response. More data is needed to see if NRT will assist the postoperative programming of the device. Comparison of more NRT measurements of individual patients in the time course may reveal in the future if NRT is able to detect movement of the electrodes out of the lateral recess. Other factors that interfere with the electrode/tissue contact surface such as tissue growth and changes caused by inflammation also may be documented or be detected earlier with this kind of electrophysiological functional neuromonitoring. Future developments of the measurement software might help to determine the optimal stimulation rate and an objective measure of channel interaction and neural excitation spread.

Together with electrically evoked auditory brainstem response (EABR) testing, neural response telemetry (NRT) may assist intraoperative placement of auditory brainstem implants (ABI) and other central auditory implants (SAI) in the future. In this study the application of intra-operative NRT in ABI is described for the first time. The recording of NRT is technically easy and does not result in prolonged operation time. When postoperative recordings are compared to intraindividual postoperative follow-up NRT measurements it may also be useful in detecting electrode movement in the clinical course.

More data is needed to determine to what degree the measurements can assess neural responsiveness of the auditory structures available and to what degree it will be useful in improving postoperative performance of ABI patients.

4.3.2. A new classification of NRT responses

0	No response	Flatline	
1	No response	Only stimulus artefact	
2	No response	Artefact rejection (XX)	
3	Questionable response	Jagged trace	
4	Questionable response	Stimulus artefact	
5	Questionable response	Skislope type, only falling pattern	
6	Biological response	Distorted, low amplitude	
7	Biological response	Typical, high amplitude	
8	Biological response	Typical, including N1	

Table 5: Intraoperative Neural Response Telemetry: Response Classification (from Kuchta et al, Fourth International conference on Vestibular schwannomas, Cambridge 2003).

To simplify the discussion about the individual responses, the following classification of NRT responses (Table 5) is suggested: A flatline response, a response rejected by the internal algorithms of the NRT program (as indicated by the "X" on the display) and a trace where only the stimulus artefact without any late component was seen was classified as "no response" (class 0-2). A jagged trace and a trace severely distorted by the early stimulus artefact so that the late components are not clearly defined was classified as a "questionable response" (class 3-4). Also traces that given a measurement delay of 50 us only showed a falling pattern without any ascending component of the potential were classified as "questionable responses" (class 5). These so called "ski-slope" responses were excluded from the analysis because the origin of the trace is not clearly biologic and may eventually represent a late artefact caused by the probe stimulus. In most cases (46,8%)

"cochlea- like" responses with the typical CAP- waveform were found after monopolar stimulation. Only these responses were considered to represent the electrically evoked compound action potential of the stimulated neurons in the cochlear nucleus. The type of the NRT responses did not correlate with the level of perceptual performance in the cases tested in chapter 3.1.1.

4.4. Discussion of laboratory studies results

Since October 2001 only studies with recordings of the central auditory pathways at the IC were performed. Stimulation was performed acoustically through the external ear or middle ear or electrically at the cochlear level. Experiments with cortical recording after stimulating the IC were not performed before October 2001. The study presented here was the first worldwide demonstrating that central stimulation of the auditory pathways is possible at the level of the IC. The stimulating current used in our experiments for IC stimulation showed thresholds that were generally lower than those used for stimulation with cochlear implants: With 200us/ phase single monopolar pulses, a median threshold of 100 uA was obtained for CI stimulation (Bierer et al, 2002). Probably because the stimulation site is closer to the stimulated neurons, the thresholds for IC stimulation were lower when compared to CI stimulation. The charge densities used for stimulation were between 1 and 10 uC/cm. According to the results of McCreery et al, 1990, this would be in a save range for the future clinical application in humans. We demonstrated a circumscribed region of low response thresholds to IC stimulation on the sylvian gyrus. The phenomenon of electrically evoked tonotopicity has been demonstrated in the early work by Woolsey and Walzl (1942) and, more recently, by Volkov and Dembnovetskii (1979) using evoked potential methodology. They were able to demonstrate a point-to-area representation of cochlear nerve fibers in the cortex. Areas of high-amplitude, short latency responses were found in dorsal and ventral AI regions. In normal hearing animals the identification of cortical recording sites is usually based on the local tonotopic gradient rather than on sulcal landmarks. The reason is that the exact position and extent of the sulcal pattern can vary substantially. In general, the cortical site with the frequency similar to the corresponding laminae within the IC ("tonotopically matched") should have the lowest threshold for stimulation. These surface recordings were refined by M.

Lenarz in 2004, who was able to show that frequency-specific activation of the IC is possible. On the basic reserch level, more studies evaluating different types of stimulation and patterns of stimulation will be following in the next years with the goal to find out more about the ideal "input" for stimulating the IC.

4.5   Conclusions regarding the clinical application of central auditory implants

Penetrating microelectrodes entail additional risks beyond those of the present ABI electrodes. Many patients with the surface electrode ABI report little change in pitch across the electrodes. We suspect that this lack of pitch change will not be a problem with penetrating microelectrodes that access the tonotopic axis of the central auditory pathways in a more localized fashion. Physiological results with penetrating microelectrodes in the cochlear nucleus of cats (McCreery et al., 1997) have demonstrated a stimulus induced depression of neural excitability (SIDNE). This depression of excitability becomes quite severe at pulse rates of 500 Hz and faster, and the depression can last for many days following termination of stimulation. No evidence of SIDNE was found based on the data of the first clinical PABI patients presented here.

At the present time it seems that with multichannel electrical stimulation of the human cochlear nucleus we are not able to produce a performance comparable to that seen in cochlear implants. It is not clear if we are not stimulating the CN in a meaningful tonotopic pattern, or because essential intrinsic processing in the CN is bypassed. Penetrating microelectrode stimulation (CN or IC) may overcome some, but not all of these potential limitations. If the limiting factor in ABI performance is that the surface electrode is stimulating the wrong subunit of the CN and/or stimulating in a nontonotopic manner, then a penetrating microelectrode could overcome these problems by stimulating the VCN locally and tonotopically.   If the limiting factor is that direct electrical stimulation bypasses or interferes with intrinsic neural processing, then the same limitation might apply to penetrating electrodes in the CN and even more to stimulation in higher centers such as the IC.

The SAI has much further implications and indications than the "common" ABI system. It can be of benefit for a much brouder group of patients. All patients deafened from Neurofibromatosis Type 2,   Aplasia or Dysplasia of the cochlea, temporal bone trauma or other bilateral lesions of the vestibulocochlear nerve and/ or the cochlea (malformations, ossification, fibrosis) may be possible candidates for SAI implantation. In these patients, it is virtually impossible or non-functional to insert a cochlear electrode. Hearing loss after severe head trauma may involve any level of the auditory pathways (conductive/ mixed/ sensorineural). 8% of these patients suffer from severe or profound bilateral impairment (Coletti et al 2004). Cochlear implants have been of little or no use in these patients.

In the Verona group, 9 patients deafened by cochlear ossification, 5 patients after head injury, 3 patients with cochlear nerve avulsion, 1 patient with auditory neuropathy and 3 patients with cochlear aplasia received auditory brainstem implants (Colletti et al 2003). Post-implant perceptual performance results in these non-tumor patients were much better when compared to the tumor (NF2) patients as reported in the previous chapters. These results of ABI implantation are very motivating for the developement of non--invasive central auditory implants. Risks and possible complications of SAI implantation include haemorrhage, infection and possibly induction of seizures. Based on the experience with deep brain implantation for movement disorders, the risk for such events is between 1-4%. In the Cologne series the incidence of intracranial bleedings associated with deep brain electrode implantation has been reduced to 0.6%. A malfunction of the receiver/stimulator device or a wrong placement of the electrodes are other possible complications. Other non-auditory side effects (NASE/ chapter 2.8.1.) may occur depending on the intracranial structures beeing stimulated. These reversible events must be contrasted to the expected benefit for the patients, which is the restoration of useful hearing in a situation of complete deafness.

For minimally invasive stereotactic auditory implantation also patients who were operated on their vestibular schwannomas when or where the implantation of an ABI was not available may qualify. Due to the minimized operative trauma, the SAI implantation may be indicated in much more patients where restoration of hearing was not an option up to now.

5.   Summary

Introduction:

Patients who became deaf due to bilateral retrocochlear lesions such as vestibular schwannomas do not benefit from mechanical hearing aids or cochlear implants. At the House

Ear Institute (HEI), Los Angeles, the auditory brainstem implant (ABI) has been developed for implantation close to the cochlear nucleus (CN) to provide some degree of hearing for these patients. Developments in microelectronics and stereotactic neurosurgery now allow also minimally invasive approaches and other targets for implantation along the central auditory pathways. The evaluation of the ABI implantations up to now and the development of alternatives is the aim of this study.

Methods:

During a one-year stay as a research fellow at the House Ear Institute, Los Angeles, 129 ABI implantations were analyzed in a retrospective study. A SPSS database was established including all available clinical, audiological, radiological and surgical data. Using this database, the resultant perceptual performance and non-auditory side-effects were analyzed for the first time. Individual clinical, radiological and surgical factors were analyzed concerning their contribution to speech perception.

The first functional intraoperative neuromonitoring with Neural Response Telemetry (NRT) was performed during this study in n=7 ABI patients intraoperatively and N=17 patients postoperatively. The analysis of postoperative electrode positions (based on postoperative MRI scans in 46 ABI patients) revealed non-auditory side-effects in relation to electrode positions. Together with Bill Hitselberger, the first deep brain implantation of a penetrating ABI (PABI) in combination with a conventional surface ABI was performed in a cadaver head via the translabyrinthine approach. In acute animal studies at the Epstein Laboratory/ University of California at San Francisco, penetrating deep-brain electrode implantations were performed in the inferior colliculus (IC) of a cat. The cortical potentials in response to electrical stimulation at the IC were recorded and analyzed. In collaboration with the Med-el company, Innsbruck based on the results mentioned above, a deep-brain electrode prototype for minimally invasive stereotactic implantation into the IC was developed. The general aim in the development of central neuroprosthesis as presented here is an improvement of speech recognition by optimizing the soft and hardware as well as the evaluation of new targets and minimally invasive approaches. One idea of this interdisciplinary study is to apply the technique of stereotactic deep-brain implantation for parkinsons disease to targets along the central auditory pathway.

Results:

Intraoperative neuromonitoring with neural response telemetry (NRT) in ABI, as presented here for the first time provides information about the postoperative perceptual performance on the basis of the intraoperative waveforms. A classification of these waveforms is presented here for the first time. The analysis of the pitch ratings in the 129 ABI patients examined here showed that significant frequency information can be perceived in spite of the reduced access to the three-dimensional structure in ABI stimulation. A wider pitch range was correlated with better results in CUNY-sentence recognition. For the recognition of vocals and single MTS-words no clear correlation was found. Non-auditory side effects (NASE) under ABI stimulation occured mainly ipsilateral and were sensoric in most cases. Motoric side effects (facial nerve associated side-effects/ FASE) occured in only 6.9% of patients at initial stimulation ("hook-up") and disapperared in the following weeks due to reprogramming in nearly all cases. Concerning the postoperative position of the ABI (based on N=46 ABI patients with postoperative MRI scans), the best performance scores were found with electrode positions at the entrance of the lateral recess of the 4th ventricle in contact to the ventral part of the cochlear nucleus (VCN). Positions deep inside the lateral recess or too far looking out of the recess were correlated with suboptimal performance score in all performance tests. The electrodes showed a high grade of positional stability in the follow-up between 6 weeks and up to 8 years postoperatively (n=129 ABI patients). A big/huge lateral recess as assessed on the preoperative MRI was correlated with subaverage performance and an increased rate of electrode dislocation. 6 of the 129 patients underwent preoperative stereotactic irradiation for the treatment of their vestibular schwannomas. Perceptual performance in these patients was subaverage but satisfying test scores were achieved in some patients, specially when the intraoperative EABR responses were preserved. Thereby preoperative stereotactic radiosurgery should not be considered as a contraindication for ABI implantation any more. The number of functional ABI electrodes did not correlate significantly with hearing performance in most tests. With three individual channels (i.e. electrodes), good results were achieved in vocal (>30%), consonant (>10%) and MTS-word (>40%) recognition. For above-average performance in open sentence recognition (CUNY-sentence recognition >10%), eight functional channels were advantageous.

The first implantation of a penetrating deep-brain electrode (PABI) into the cochlear nucleus in a cadaver specimen demonstrated the adequate design of the electrode and the developed applicator tool. The simultaneous implantation of PABI and surface-ABI electrode is feasible after microsurgical removal of a vestibular schwannoma via the translab approach. We were also able to perform postoperative MRI and CT imaging of the implanted PABI electrode for the first time. The prototype multichannel deep-brain electrode for stereotactic implantation (SAI) into the IC that has been developed within this project, has a diameter of 1.27mm and consists of a silicon carrier with 12 plate electrodes. A Nitinol mandrin within the electrode carrier provides directional stability during stereotactic application of the SAI device. The minimally invasive stereotactic frontal-transcerebral approach that was developed specially for SAI implantation provides maximal stability of the electrode with minimal risk for eloquent brain regions.

Conclusions:

Based on the data of 129 implanted patients, the ABI proved to be of invaluable benefit over a period of more than 8 years, with evidence of continual improvement in performance over time. Nonauditory sensations, when they occur, could be eliminated or reduced by proper selection of stimulation parameters and/or switching off individual electrodes. In spite of the apparently inappropriate and non-tonotopic electrode position in vicinity of the cochlear nucleus, the present surface electrode system is beneficial in patients deafened by bilateral vestibular schwannomas. ABI patients receive significant improvement in lipreading, and can distinguish sounds on the basis of temporal envelope cues. One reason for the surprisingly good speech perception results of surface-ABI implantation at the level of the CN is the high plasticity and pattern recognition ability of the human brain. Even reduced or distorted acoustic informantion will be recognized by the patient if this information has made its way from the CN and the IC to the auditory cortex. Specially sound effects (cars, doorbell...) are identified easily by most (118 out of 129) ABI patients on the basis of the amplitude envelope. Minimally invasive stereotactic SAI-implantation as presented here for the first time would be an alternative to restore a significant amount of hearing for thousands of patients in which an open neurosurgical operation is not indicated (non-tumor patients). Patients who have lost their hearing due to diseases such as cochlear ossification, head injuries, temporal bone fractures, auditory neuropathy and cochlear aplasia may become possible candidates for central auditory implantation. The direct access to the three-dimensional tonotopy of the structures stimulated may result in perceptual performance levels even above those achieved with surface-ABI stimulation.

6. Zusammenfassung

Einführung:

Patienten, die auf Grund einer beidseitigen retrocochleären Erkrankung z.b. durch ein Akkustikusneurinom ertaubt sind haben nicht die Möglichkeit der Hörrehabilitation durch mechanische Hörhilfen oder ein Cochleaimplantat. Vor 25 Jahren wurde im House-Ear Institute (HEI) in Los Angeles erstmals im Rahmen einer neurochirurgisch- HNO-ärztlichen Kooperation eine Elektrode in die Nähe des Nucleus Cochlearis (CN) implantiert. Der CN liegt im Hirnstamm und stellt die Eintrittspforte für die akustischen Information ins Gehirn dar. Entwicklungen auf dem Gebiet der Mikroelektronik sowie der stereotaktischen Neurochirurgie ermöglichen jedoch auch weitere minimal- invasive Implantationsmethoden und weitere Implantationsziele entlang der zentralen Hörbahn. Die Evaluation der durchgeführten Hirnstammimplantationen mit dem Ziel der Weiterentwicklung der zentralen Hörprothetik und der Entwicklung von Alternativen ist das Ziel dieser Arbeit.

Methodik:

Im Rahmen eines einjährigen Forschungsaufenthalts am House Ear Institute, Los Angeles wurden die bisherigen ABI Implantationen im Rahmen einer retrospektiven Studie analysiert. Es wurde eine SPSS Datenbank mit allen klinischen, audiologischen, radiologischen und chirurgischen Daten etabliert. Mit Hilfe dieser Datenbank konnten nun erstmals die resultierenden Hörergebnisse unter Stimulation sowie alle Nebenwirkungen analysiert werden. Individuelle klinische, radiologische und chirurgische Faktoren konnten jetzt erstmals im Hinblick auf ihren Einfluss auf das Hörergebnis untersucht werden.

Parallel dazu wurde erstmals intraoperativ die Anwendung des klinischen Monitorings durch Neural Response Telemetry (NRT) bei sieben ABI Implantationen untersucht. 99 NRT Ableitungen wurden erstmals in 17 ABI Patienten postoperativ abgeleitet. Eine Analyse der postoperativen Elektrodenpositionen im MRT zeigt Nebenwirkungen der Stimulation in Abhängigkeit von der Elektrodenlage. Zur Vorbereitung der erstmaligen klinischen Tiefenhirnimplantation wurde in Zusammenarbeit mit William Hitselberger am HEI

Implantationen über den translabyrinthären Zugang am Leichenpräparat durchgeführt und ausgewertet. Im Rahmen eines Akutversuches im Epstein Labor für Neurologische Forschung an der Universität von San Francisco wurde eine Tiefenhirn-Elektrodenimplantation im Colliculus i nferior einer Katze durchgeführt. Die resultierenden Antwortpotentiale wurden cortikal durch Mikroelektroden abgeleitet.

In Zusammenarbeit mit der Firma Med-El/ Innsbruck wurde basierend auf den Ergebnissen der oben beschriebenen Studien eine Tiefenhirnelektrode zur stereotaktischen Implantation in den Inferior Colliculus entwickelt. Allgemeines Ziel der Weiterentwicklung von zentralen Hörprothesen ist die Verbesserung des Sprachverständnisses durch Optimierung der Soft,- und Hardware, sowie durch Evaluation neuer Zielstrukturen und minimal invasiver Zugangswege. Das spezielle Ziel der hier dargestellten Arbeiten ist die Entwicklung und erstmalige Anwendung von minimal-invasiven Implantationsmethoden für die Stimulation der zentralen Hörbahn. Es handelt sich um eine interdisziplinäre neurochirurgisch/ hals-nasen-ohren-ärztliche Studie mit dem Ziel, die Technik der stereotaktischen Tiefenhirnstimulation, wie sie aus der Therapie des Morbus Parkinson bekannt ist, auf Schaltstellen der zentralen Hörbahn anzuwenden.

Ergebnisse:

Die im Rahmen dieser Arbeit erstmals bei auditorischen Hirnstammimplantaten angewandte Technik des intraoperativen Neuromonitorings mit Neural Response Telemetry (NRT) erlaubt durch Analyse der erhaltenen Wellenformen Aussagen über das postoperative Hörergebnis des Implantates. Im Rahmen der Arbeit wird eine neue Klassifikation der NRT Wellenformen bei ABI vorgestellt. Die Analyse des "Pitch ratings" der 129 untersuchten ABI Patienten zeigte dass signifikante Frequenzinformationen trotz eingeschränkter Erreichbarkeit der dreidimensionalen Struktur bei Oberflächenstimulation des CN wahrgenommen werden können. Eine grösseres Frequenzspektrum ("Pitch range") des ABI Implantates korrelierte deutlich mit höheren Testergebnissen bei der Satzerkennung (CUNY sentences). Für das Erkennen von Konsonanten, Vokalen und einzelnen Wörtern (MTS-Word-test) fand sich keine signifikante Abhängigkeit. Bei der Analyse der auftretenden Nebenwirkungen fanden sich vorwiegend ipsilaterale Reizsensationen im Gesichtsbereich unter Stimulation. Motorische Nebenwirkungen (Facial Nerve associated side-effects, FASE) fanden sich bei initialer Stimulation in 6,9% der Patienten bei initialer Stimulation und spielten im Langzeitverlauf durch Reprogrammierung des Generators keine Rolle mehr. Bei der Korrelation der

Hörergebnisse mit der postoperativen Position der Implantate, analysiert anhand von MRT Bildern (N=46), zeigten sich die besten "performance scores" bei ABI Positionierung im Eingangsbereich des vierten Ventrikels in Kontakt zu dem ventralen Anteil des Nucleus Cochlearis (VCN). Sehr tief im lateralen Rezessus oder zu weit aus dem Rezessus plazierte Elektroden zeigten in allen Qualitäten signifikant schlechtere Hörergebnisse.

Die Elektroden zeigten radiologisch und funktionell (Stimulierbarkeit der einzelnen Elektroden) einen hohen Grad von Ortsstabilität im Zeitraum zwischen 6 Wochen und bis zu 8 Jahren postoperativ (n=129 ABI Patienten). Patienten mit einem durch Tumor oder anlagebedingt deutlich vergrösserten lateralen Rezessus zeigten deutlich schlechtere Hörergebnisse und eine grössere Tendenz zur Dislokation.

6 der insgesamt 129 in der Datenbank erfassten ABI Patienten wurden präoperativ zur Behandlung der Akkustikusneurinome stereotaktisch bestrahlt. Die Hörergebnisse nach stereotaktischer Bestrahlung des Hörnerven sind unterdurchschnittlich, es lassen sich jedoch insbesondere bei intraoperativ erhaltener EABR Antwort befriedigende Hörergebnisse erreichen. Insofern stellt eine vorangehende radiochirurgische Behandlung keine Kontraindikation für die ABI Implantation mehr dar. Die Anzahl der funktionellen ABI Elektroden korrelierte beim Oberflächen-ABI nicht signifikant mit den Ergebnissen der Hörtests. Mit mindestens drei individuell programmierten Stimulationskanälen (i.e.: Elektroden) liessen sich befriedigende Ergebnisse bei Vokal- (>30%), Konsonant (>10%) und MTS-Worterkennung (>40%) erreichen. Für das freie Verständnis von gesprochenen Sätzen (CUNY sentence recognition > 10%) waren jedoch 8 Kanäle oder mehr vorteilhaft. Die im HEI in Rahmen dieser Arbeit erstmals durchgeführte Implantation einer penetrierenden Tiefenhirnelektrode (PABI) im Nucleus Cochlearis einer präparierten Leiche zeigte das adäquate Design des Applikationsinstrumentes für den translabyrinthinen (TL) Zugang. Die Implantation einer PABI und einer Oberflächen-ABI Elektrode im Rahmen einer AN-Tumorentfernung ist praktisch möglich. Im Rahmen dieser Arbeit wurde auch erstmals weltweit eine postoperative CCT und MRT Bildgebung nach PABI Implantation durchgeführt. Der im letzten Teil dieser Arbeit entwickelte Prototyp einer Mehrkanal-Tiefenhirnelektrode zur stereotaktischen Implantation in den Colliculus Inferior besteht aus einem Silikonträger mit einem Durchmesser von 1,27mm, auf dem 12 Plättchenelektroden angebracht sind. Im Inneren der nadelförmigen Mehrkanalelektrode sorgt ein Nitinolmandrin für Richtungsstabilität bei der stereotaktischen Implantation. Der an Hand von computerisierten MRT- Aufnahmen entwickelte minimal invasive frontal-transcerebrale

stereotaktische Zugang zum Mittelhirn sorgt für eine maximale Stabilität der implantierten SAI-Elektrode bei minimaler Gefährdung von eloquenten Hirnregionen. Durch das durchgeführte Tierexperiment wurde erstmals gezeigt, dass die Stimulation der zentralen Hörbahn durch IC-Elektroden möglich ist. Die kortikal abgeleitete Stimulationsantwort ist Vorraussetzung für das angestrebte Sprachverständnis in der zukünftigen klinischen Anwendung.

Schlussfolgerungen:

Die Analyse der audiologischen Testergebnisse von 129 implantierten Patienten mit dem 21-Kanal Nucleus Hirnstammimplantat zeigt, dass obwohl der in Kontakt zur Oberfläche des Nucleus cochlearis (CN) implantierte Elektrodenträger nur einen sehr reduzierten Zugriff auf die verschiedenen Frequenzen in der Tiefe des CN erlaubt, in den meisten implantierten Patienten ein befriedigendes alltagsrelevantes Hörergebnis erzielt wird. Durch Re-Programmierung und Lernvorgänge steigern sich die Hörergebnisse über mehr als acht Jahre kontinuierlich. Ein Grund für die überraschend guten Hörergebnisse bei Stimulation der Oberfläche des CN ist die Plastizität des menschlichen Gehirns. Auch reduzierte und verzerrte Informationen, die den Weg über eine implantierte Elektrode in den CN, den Inferior Colliculus und schliesslich den auditorischen Kortex finden, werden nach monatelangem Training als sinnvolle Höreindrücke wahrgenommen. Eine hier erstmals vorgestellt stereotaktische Implantationsmöglichkeit würde für mehrere Tausend Patienten bei denen eine offene, neurochirurgische Operation nicht in Frage kommt, eine neue Möglichkeit zur Wiederherstellung eines alltagsrelevanten Hörvermögens darstellen. Darüber hinaus ist durch direkteren Zugriff auf die frequenzselektiven Areale der zentralen Hörbahn bei der stereotaktischen "deep brain" Implantation ein besseres Hörergebnis im Vergleich zu den bisher existierenden ABI-Oberflächenelektroden zu erwarten.

7.   Acknowledgements

Behr, Robert (Prof. Dr. med., Chairman of the Department of Neurosurgery, Städtisches Klinikum Fulda): for beeing the first who introduced me to ABI technique and implantation; for infecting me with the idea of central auditory implants; for supporting my grant application , for editing this manuscript and supplying invaluable ideas.

Jolly, Claude (Ph.D., Director of Electrode Developement, Med-El Company, Innsbruck, Austria): for beeing open to my design of the SAI electrode and giving me the chance to participate in his experience concerning electrode development.

Kade, Max foundation and DFG (in the person of Mr. Frank Grünhagen, DFG, Bonn): for beeing open to my ideas and providing the financial background to spent one year at HEI in Los Angeles.

Klug, Norfrid (Prof. Dr. med., Chairman of the Department of Neurosurgery, Cologne University): for beeing my teacher in general neurosurgery over more than 10 years at my "second home", the Department of Neurosurgery at Cologne University; for indispensible long-time paternal support, confidence, and motivation during ten years of my clinical and scientific life.

Linke, Detlef Bernhard (Prof. Dr. med., Chairman of the Department of Clinical Neurorehablitation and Clinical Neurophysiology, Bonn University): for demonstrating me how to address really important questions and how to keep on struggling although there are no answers to these questions; for beeing a role-model in developing an individual style in neurosciences; for introducing me to scientific thinking, the mind-body problem and clinical electrophysiology.

McCreery, Douglas ("Dough") (Ph.D. Director of the Neural Engineering Program, Huntington Memorial Research Institute, Pasadena, CA, USA): for spending days and nights in my car and in the lab; for our overnight trips to Chris Schreiner in San Francisco; nobody knows more about microelectrodes and about what´s happening in the brain of a cat.

Otto, Steve (M.A., Audiologist, Clinical Coordinator of the ABI program at HEI): for becoming a friend; nobody in the world knows more about testing and programming an ABI; for showing me how combining music and medicine makes sense for the patient and the professional.

Schreiner, Christof ("Chris") (M.D., Ph-D. Keck Center for Integrative Neuroscience and department of Otolaryngology, University of California at San Francisco) for spending days and nights with me and Dough in his lab to see what happens when we stimulate the IC.

Shannon, Robert ("Bob") (Ph.D., Chairman of the Department of Auditory Implants and Perception (DAIP), House Ear Institute HEI), Los Angeles, USA): for beeing the ideal director of a clinical and research unit; always open ears and (literally!) open doors for his residents and partners; for the best strawberry margaritas in the world and the best year of my life so far.

Sturm, Volker (Prof. Dr. med., Chairman of the Departement of Stereotaxy and Functional Neurosurgery, Cologne University): for beeing my teacher from 1995-1996; for beeing open to innovative ideas and approaches; for teaching me what modern minimally invasive neurosurgery is about.

8.   Glossary

-**Audiology** : the measurement of hearing (syn: audiometry)

-**Auditory**: of or pertaining to hearing, or to the sense or organs of hearing

-**Auditory brainstem implant (ABI)**: a prosthetic device that provides auditory information to the brainstem (the area where the auditory nerve enters the brain)

-**Averaging**: to find the mean of, when sums or quantities are unequal; to reduce to a mean.

-**Brainstem**: the part of the brain continuous with the spinal cord and comprising the medulla oblongata

-**CUNY** (City University of New York Sentences, Tyler/Preece et al 1987) sentence recognition Test; standardized video test on a laser disk that tests open-speech sentence recognition in the sound-only condition.

-**Compound action potential (cCAP)**: (compound= consisting of two or more substances or ingredients or elements or parts; composed of many distinct individuals united to form a whole) near-field potentials summarizing the activity from a group of nerve cells (here: activity within the cochlear nucleus after electrical stimulation via the ABI)

-**EABR**: Electrically evoked auditory brainstem responses; response evoked by electrical stimulation of the cochlear nucleus and recorded from the skin. EABR has become the gold standart for intraoperative neuromonitoring in ABI implantation. EABR can demonstrate appropriate electrode placement and system integrity. Recording electrodes are placed at the vertex (Cz) and over C7 at the neck.

-**Electrode**: a conductor used to make electrical contact with some part of a circuit

-**Electromyography (EMG)**: Here: intraoperative monitoring of the neural integrity of the eleventh and ninth cranial nerves by measuring the spontaneous activity of the corresponding musces

-**HEI (House Ear Institute)**: largest research institute and clinic concerning hearing disorders in the world, located in Los Angeles, California, USA. The cochlear implant and the auditory implant have been developed here.

-**Intelligibility**: the quality of language that is comprehensible

-**Loudness**: the magnitude of sound (usually in a specified direction)

-**MTS** word recognition test: "Monosyllable, Spondee, Trochee" (MTS) test; consists of 12 words that differ in the number of syllables (monosyllable vs. others) and in the stress patterns in two-syllable words (spondee vs. trochee); results are evaluated both in terms of stress patterns correct and number of words correct

-**Neural response telemetry (NRT)**: bi-directional telemetric system/ radio-frequency pulses are transmitted from the speech processor interface across the skin barrier to the implanted receiver/stimulator device. The responses to stimulation were averaged, analyzed and the resultant CAP waveform is displayed on a computer.

-**Pitch**: the property of sound that varies with variation in the frequency of vibration

-**Pitch range test**: the subjective pitch of the auditory percepts on each useable electrode was assessed on a visual analog scale ranging from 1(lowest pitch) to 100 (highest pitch). Ten judgements were obtained per electrode, which yielded an estimate of the range and variability of pitch percepts and suggested the degree to which electrodes may have been activating different neural populations. The overall pitch range was defined as the range from the lowest to the highest subjective pitch sensation on the visual analog scale (1-100). When all stimulated channels had the same pitch, or the patient was unable to assess the pitch level, the overall pitch range was 0.

-**Prosthesis**: corrective consisting of a replacement for a part of the body; called also prothesis

-**Prosthetic**: of or relating to prosthetics; relating to or serving as a prosthesis

-**Receiver**: set that receives radio or tv signals (here: radiofrequency coded auditory information transmitted through the skin from the external speech processor)

-**Range**: an area in which something acts or operates or has power or control; the limits within which something can be effective

-**Ratio**: the relative magnitudes of two quantities (usually expressed as a quotient)

-**Sound effect recognition test (SERT)**: is a four-alternative test of environmental sound discrimination with chance performance level of 25%. Single nonspeech sound are not matched in their temporal patterns or frequency content, so that identification of their temporal pattern alone may allow correct identification

-**Spectrum**: an ordered array of the components of an emission or wave; broad range of related values or qualities or ideas or activities
-**Speech**: the act of delivering a formal spoken communication to an audience; communication by word of mouth; something spoken; the exchange of spoken words

-**Speech tests**: The vowel, consonant and CUNY sentence tests were presented in sound-only, vision-only and sound-plus-vision modes. All other tests were administered in sound-only mode. A single male talker produced both vowels and consonants. Constant confusion matrices were compiled from five presentations of 16 medial consonants (ama, ana, afa, etc.) for each listener. Vowel confusions matrices were compiled from three presentations of 8 vowels in a h/V/d context (heed, hid, had, etc.). Chance performance level of the consonant recognition test was 7.14% correct and the 95% confidence level was 11.1% correct.

-**Telemetry**: automatic transmission and measurement of data from remote sources by wire or radio or other means

-**Warping**: to throw; hence, to send forth, or throw out; to turn or twist out of shape

9. References

Baser ME., Ragge NK, et al.: Phenotypic variability in monozygotic twins with neurofibromatosis 2. Am J Med Genet 64(4): 563-7, 1996.

Behr R, Hofmann E.: Magnetic resonance imaging (MRI) in patients with implanted ABI (Combi 40+): Experience in 5 cases. Wiener Medizinische Wochenschrift 156 (119):45, 2006.

Behr R, Mueller J, Shehata-Dieler W, Schlake HP, Helms J, Roosen K, Klug N, Hölper B, Lorens A: The High Rate CIS Auditory Brainstem Implant for Restoration of Hearing in NF-2 Patients. Skull Base 17; 91-107;, Presentation at the 9th Congress of the European Skull Base Society, Prague, 2007..

Behr R. Experiences and results with auditory brainstem implants (ABI) in NF-2 patients. Klin Neurophysiol 37; 1055: 939097, 2006.

Behr R, Mark G, Bartik H, Hölper B: Bilateral Electrical Stimulation of the Cochlar Nucleus: Surgical and Technical Feasibility. Skull Base 16, 1055; 957295, 2006.

Benabid AL: Deep brain stimulation for Parkinson´s disease. Curr Opin Neurobiol 13(6)696-706, 2003.

Benabid K, Wallace B, Bell BA, Benabid AL: Deep brain stimulation of the subthalamic nucleus in Parkinson´s disease 1993-2003: where are we 10 years on? Br J Neurosurg 18(1):19-38, 2004.

Bierer JA, Middlebrooks JC: Auditory cortical images of cochlear- implant stimuli: dependence on electrode configuration. J Neurophysiol 87:478-92, 2002.

Bijlsma, EK, Merel P, et al.: Family with neurofibromatosis type 2 and autosomal dominant hearing loss: identification of carriers of the mutated NF2 gene. Hum Genet 96(1): 1-5, 1995.

Blamey PJ, Pyman BC et al.: Factors predicting postoperative sentence scores in postlingually deaf adult cochlear implant patients. Annals of Otology, Rhinology and Laryngology, 101, 342-348, 1992.

Boex CS, Eddington DE, Noel VA, Rabinowitz WM, Tierney J, and Whearty ME: Restoration of normal loudness growth for CIS sound coding strategies, Abstracts of the 1997 Conference on Implantable Auditory Prostheses, Asilomar, CA, August, page 26, 1997.

Brackmann DE, Hitselberger W, Nelson RA, Moore JK, Waring M, Portillo F, Shannon RV, and Telischi F.: Auditory Brainstem Implant. I: Issues in Surgical Implantation, Otolaryngology, Head and Neck Surgery, 108, 624-634, 1993.

Brackmann DE, Fayad JN, Slattery WH 3rd, Friedman RA, Day JD, Hitselberger WE, Owens RM: Early proactive management of vestibular schwannomas in neurofibromatosis type 2. Neurosurgery 49(2):274-80, 2001.

Bredberg G. and Lindstrom B: Insertion length of electrode array and its relation to speech communication performance and nonauditory side effects in multichannel-implanted patients. Annals of Otology, Rhinology and Laryngology, Suppl. 166, 256-258, 1995.

Brill S: Optimization of channel number and stimulation rate in the COMBI 40+, International Workshop on Cochlear Implants, Vienna, Austria, October 24-25, 1996.

Brown CJ, Abbas bPJ, Fryauf-Bertschy H, Kelsay D, Gantz BJ: Intraoperative and postoperative electrically evoked auditory brain stem responses in nucleus cochlear implant users: implications for the fitting process. Ear Hear 15:168-176, 1994.

Brown CJ, Abbas PJ, Gantz B: Electrically evoked whole-nerve action potentials: data from human cochlear implant users. J Acoust Soc Am 88:1385-1391, 1990.

Chatterjee M. and Shannon RV: Forward masking excitation patterns as a measure of electrode interaction in cochlear implants: dependence on stimulus parameters. Journal of the Acoustical Society of America, 103(5), 1998.

Cohen LT, Busby PA, Whitford LA and Clark GM: Cochlear implant place psychophysics: 1. Pitch estimation with deeply inserted electrodes, Audiology & Neuro-Otology, 1, 265-277, 1996a.

Cohen LT, Busby PA and Clark GM: Cochlear implant place psychophysics: 2. Comparison of forward masking and pitch estimation data, Audiology & Neuro-Otology, 1, 278-292, 1996b.

Colletti V, Fiorino F, Sacchetto L, et al: Hearing habilitation with auditory brainstem implantation in two children with cochlear nerve aplasia.   Int J Pediatr Otorhinolaryngol 60:99-111, 2001.

Colletti V, Fiorino FG, Carner M, et al: The retrosigmoid approach for auditory brainstem implantation. Am J Otol 21:826-836, 2000.

Colletti V, Sacchetto L, Giarbini N, et al: Retrosigmoid approach for auditory brainstem implant. J Laryngol Otol 114 (Suppl 27):37-40, 2000.

Colletti V, Fiorino F, Carner M, et al: Hearing habilitation with auditory brainstem implantation in two children with cochlear nerve aplasia. Int J Ped Otorhinlo 60:99-111, 2001.

Colletti V, Fiorino F, Carner M, et al: Auditory brainstem implantation: The university of Verona experience. Otolaryngol Head Neck Surg 127: 84-96, 2002.

Colletti V, Fiorino F, Carner M, et al: Auditory brainstem implant (ABI): New frontiers in adults and children. Otol Neurotol, in press.

Colletti V, Carner M, Miorelli V, Colletti L, Guida M, Fiorino F: Auditory brainstem implant in posttraumatic cochlear nerve avulsion. Audiol Neurotol 9:247-255, 2004.

Colletti V, Shannon RV: Open set speech perception with auditory brainstem implants? Laryngoscope 115:1974-1987, 2005.

Colletti V, Shannon RV, Carner M, Colletti L: First successful case of electrical stimulation of the human inferior colliculus. Wiener Medizinische Wochenschrift 156 (119):45, 2006.

Colletti V: State of the Art of Auditory Brainstem Implants. Skull Base 17: 1055; 984018, Presentation at the 9th Congress of the European Skull Base Society, Prague, 2007.

Collins LM, Zwolan TA and Wakefield GH: Comparison of electrode discrimination, pitch ranking, and pitch scaling in postlingually deafened adult cochlear implant subjects, J. Acoust. Soc. Amer., 1998.

Cushing H: Tumors of the Nervus Acusticus and the Syndrome of the Cerebellopontine Angle,   Philadelphia and London: W.B. Saunders Co; 1917.

Daniloff RG, Shiner TH and Zemlin WR: Intelligibility of vowels altered in duration and frequency, J. Acoust. Soc. Amer., 44, 700-707, 1968.

Delhorne LA, Eddington DE, Noel VA, Rabinowitz WM, Tierney J and Whearty ME: Speech reception with CIS processing: Longitudinal evaluations and implications from acoustic simulations, Abstracts of the 1997 Conference on Implantable Auditory Prostheses, Asilomar, CA, August, page 49, 1997.

Deuschl G, Bain P: Deep brain stimulation for tremor: patient selection and evaluation. Mov Disord 17, Suppl 3:102-11, 2002.

Dillier N, Lai WK, Almqvist B, Frohne C, Muller-Deile J, Stecker M, von Wallenberg E: Measurement of the electrically evoked compound action potential via a neural response telemetry system. Ann Otol Rhinol Laryngol 111:407-414, 2002.

Dorman MF, Loizou PC and Rainey D: Speech intelligibility as a function of the number of channels of stimulation for signal processors using sine-wave and noise-band outputs, J. Acoust. Soc. Amer., 102, 2403-2411, 1997a.

Dorman MF, Loizou PC and Rainey D: Simulating the effect of cochlear-implant electrode insertion-depth on speech understanding", J. Acoust. Soc. Amer., 102(5), 2993-2996, 1997b.

Dorman MF, Loizou PC and Rainey D: Speech understanding as a function of the number of channels of stimulation for processors using sine-wave and noise-band outputs. Journal of the Acoustical Society of America, 102, 2403-2411, 1997c.

Eisenberg LS, Maltan AA, Portillo F, Mobley JP, House WF: Electrical stimulation of the auditory brain stem structure in deafened adults. J Rehabil Res Dev 24(3):9-22, 1987.

Escabi MA, Miller LM, Read HL, Schreiner CE: Naturalistic auditory contrast improves spectotemporal coding in the cat inferior colliculus. J Neurosci 17;23(37): 11489-504, 2003.

Evans DG, Trueman L, et al: Genotype/phenotype correlations in type 2 neurofibromatosis (NF2): evidence for more severe disease associated with truncating mutations [published erratum appears in J Med Genet 1999 Jan;36(1):87]. J Med Genet 35(6): 450-5, 1998.

Fishman K, Shannon RV and Slattery WH: Speech recognition as a function of the number of electrodes used in the SPEAK cochlear implant speech processor, J. Speech Hear. Res., 40, 1201-1215, 1997.

Friesen LM, ShannonVB, Baskent D, Wang X. Speech recognition in noise as a function of the number of spectral channels: Comparison of acoustic hearing and cochlear implants. J Acoust Soc Am 110(2),1150-1163, 2001.

Frohne C, Matthies C, Lesinski-Schiedat A, Battmer RD, Samii M, Lenarz T: Extensive monitoring during auditory brainstem implant surgery. J Laryngol Otol Suppl (27): 11-4, 2000.

Fu QJ, Shannon RV: Recognition of spectrally degraded and frequency-shifted vowels in acoustic and electric hearing, Journal of the Acoustical Society of America, 105(3), 1999.

Fu QJ, Shannon RV, Zeng FG, Chatterjee M: Electrode interactions measured by loudness summation in cochlear implant listeners, Journal of the Acoustical Society of America, 100, 2631, 1996.

Fu QJ, Chatterjee M, Shannon RV, Zeng FG: Comparison of electrode interaction measures in multichannel cochlear implants, Assoc. for Research in Otolaryngology Midwinter Meeting, St. Petersburg, Florida, Feb. 2-7 (poster), 1997.

Fu QJ and Shannon RV: Effects of electrode location and spacing on speech recognition with the Nucleus-22 cochlear implant, Journal of the Acoustical Society of America, 104, 1998a.

Gardner WJ, Frazier CH: Bilateral acoustic neurofibromas: A clinical study and field survey of a family of five generations with bilateral deafness in thirty-eight members. Arch Neurol Psychiatr 23: 266-302, 1930.

Gutmann DH, Carey JC et. al: The Diagnostic Evaluation and Multidisciplinary Management of NF1 and NF2." JAMA 278: 51-57, 1997.

Hillenbrand J, Getty LA, Clark MJ, Wheeler K: Acoustic characteristics of American English vowels, J. Acoust. Soc. Am. 97, 3099-3111, 1995.

Hanekom JJ and Shannon RV: Place pitch discrimination and speech recognition in cochlear implant users", South African Journal of Communication Disorders, 43, 27-40, 1996.

Hamani C, Hodaie M, Lozano AM: Present and future of deep brain stimulation for refractory epilepsy. Acta Neurochir 147(3):227-9, 2002.

Hanekom JJ. and Shannon RV: Gap detection as a measure of electrode interaction in cochlear implants: implications for speech processor fitting. Submitted to Journal of the Acoustical Society of America, June 1997.

Hill FJ, McRae LP, and McClellan RP: Speech recognition as a function of channel capacity in a discrete set of channels, J. Acoust. Soc. Amer., 44, 13-18, 1968.

Hochmair I, Arnold W, Nopp P, Jolly C, Muller J, Roland P: Deep electrode insertion in cochlear implants: apical morphology, electrodes and speech perception results. Acta Otolaryngol 123(5):612-7, 2003.

Holmes A, Kemker FJ, and Merwin G: The effects of varying the number of cochlear implant electrodes on speech perception. American Journal of Otology, 8(3), 240-246, 1987.

Huttenbrink KB, Zahnert T, Jolly C, Hofmann G: Movements of cochlear implant electrodes inside the cochlea during insertion: an x-ray microscopy study. Otol Neurotol Mar;32(2):187-91, 2002.

Jackson KB, Mark G, Helms J, Mueller J, Behr R: An auditory brainstem implant system. Am J Audiol 11(2):128-33, 2002.

Kiang NY, Keithley EM, Liberman MC: The impact of auditory nerve experiments on cochlear implant design. Ann N Y Acad Sci 405:114-121, 1983.

Kileny P, Zimmerman-Phillips S, Zwolan T, and Kemink J: Effects of channel number and place of stimulation on performance with the cochlear corporation multichannel implant. American Journal of Otology, 13(2), 117-123, 1992.

Kluwe L, S Bayer et al: Identification of NF2 germ-line mutations and comparison with neurofibromatosis 2 phenotypes [published erratum appears in Hum Genet 1997 Feb;99(2):292]." Hum Genet 98(5): 534-8, 1996.

Kuchta J, Otto SR, Shannon RV, Hitselberger WE, Brackmann DE: The multichannel auditory brainstem implant: how many electrodes make sense? J Neurosurg 96(6): 1963-71, 2002.

Kuchta J, Behr R, Walger M, Michel O, Klug N: Rehabilitation of hearing and communication functions in patients with NF2. Acta Neurochir Suppl 79:109-111, 2002.

Kuchta J, Brackmann D, Hitselberger W, Shannon R, Otto SR: Speech perception and the number of spectral channels in auditory brainstem implants. Proceedings of the Fourth International Conference on Vestibular Schwannoma and other CPA lesions. Baguley D (ed.) Cambridge 13th-17th July 2003.

Kuchta J, Otto SR, Waring M, Shannon R: Intraoperative neuromonitoring with compound action potentials in auditory brainstem implants. Proceedings of the Fourth International Conference on Vestibular Schwannoma and other CPA lesions. Baguley D (ed.) Cambridge 13th-17th July 2003.

Kuchta J, Brackmann DB, Hitselberger W, Otto S, Shannon R: Side effects of CPA stimulation with Auditory Brainstem Implants. Proceedings of the Fourth International Conference on Vestibular Schwannoma and other CPA lesions. Baguley D (ed.) Cambridge 13th-17th July 2003.

Kuchta J, Otto SR, Shannon RV, Brackmann D, Hitselberger W: Speech Perception with Audiory brainstem implants: The importance of spectral cues. Proceedings of the Fourth International Conference on Vestibular Schwannoma and other CPA lesions. Baguley D (ed.) Cambridge 13th-17th July 2003.

Kuchta J: Neuroprosthetic hearing with auditory brainstem implants. Biomed Tech 49(4): 83-7, 2004.

Kuchta J: Twentifive years auditory brainstem implants: Perspectives. Acta Neurochir (47): 245-52 (Sonderheft Neuromodulation), 2007.

Kumar K, Toth C, Nath RK: Deep brain stimulation for intractable pain: a 15 year experience. Neurosurgery 40(4):736-46, 1997.

Kumar K, Wyant GM, Nath R: Deep brain stimulation for control of intractable pain in humans, present and future: a ten-year follow up. Neurosurgery 26(5):774-81, 1990.

Lai WK, Dillier N: A simple two-component model of the electrically evoked compound action potential in the human cochlea. Audiol Neurootol 5:333-345, 2000.

Lavielle JP, Meller R, Deveze A, Tardivet L, Magnan J: Auditory Brainstem Implant with Contralateral Cochlear Implant or Serviceable Hearing. Skull Base 17; 1055: 984016, Skull Base 17, Presentation at the 9th Congress of the European Skull Base Society, Prague, 2007..

Lawson D, Wilson B, Finley C: New processing strategies for multichannel cochlear prostheses. In J.A. Allum, D.J. Allum-Mecklenburg, F.P. Harris, and R. Probst (Eds.), Natural and Artificial Control of Hearing and Balance, (pp. 313-321), Progress in Brain Research, vol. 97, Amsterdam: Elsevier, 1993.

Lenarz M, Matthies C, Lesinski-Schiedat A, Frohne C, ROst U, Illg A, Battmer RD, Samii, Lenarz T: Auditory brainstem implant part II: subjective assessment of functional outcome. Otol Neurotol 23(5):694-7, 2002.

Lenarz M, Reuter G, Patrick J, Lim H, Samii M, Lenarz T: Concept electrophysiological assessment and safety studies of the Auditory Midbrain Implant (AMI), Wiener Medizinische Wochenschrift 156 (119):44, 2006.

Lenarz T, Moshrefi M, Matthies C, Frohne C, Lesinski-Schiedat A, Illg A, Rost U, Battmer RD, Samii M: Auditory brainstem implant:part I. Auditory performance and its evolution over time. Otol Neurotol 22(6):823-33, 2001.

Lenarz T, Lim HH, Reuter G, Patrick JF, Lenarz M: The auditory midbrain implant: a new auditory prosthesis for neural deafness- concept and device description. Otol Neurotol :840-845, 2005.

Lenarz T, Samii M, Matthies C, Lesinski-Schiedat A, Battmer RD, Lenarz M: Auditory Rehabilitation with Cochlear Implants, Auditory Brainstem Implants and Auditory Midbrain Implants- A new Field for the Skull Base Surgeon. Skull Base 15; 1055: Presentation at the 7th Congress of the European Skull Base Society, Fulda, 2005.

Lesinski-Schiedat A, Frohne C, Illg A, Rost U, Matthies C, Battmer RD, Samii M, Lenarz T: Auditory brainstem implant in auditory rehabilitation of patients with neurofibromatosis type 2: Hannover programme. J Laryngol Otol Suppl (27):15-7, 2000.

Levitt H: Transformed up-down methods in psychoacoustics, J. Acoust. Soc. Amer., 49, 467-477, 1971.

Lim HH, Tong YC, Clark GM: Forward masking patterns produced by intracochlear stimulation of one and two electrode pairs in the human cochlea, J. Acoust. Soc. Am., 86, 971-980, 1989.

Lim HH, Anderson DJ: Auditory Cortical Responses to Electrical Stimulation of the Inferior Colliculus: Implications for an Auditory Midbrain Implant. J Neurophysiol 96:975-988, 2006.

Lorens A, Skaryski H, Behr R, Szuchnik J, Mrowka M, Piotrowska A: Hearing Perception of Auditory Brainstem Implanted Patient: Long-Term Results. Skull Base 15; 1055: 916405, Presentation at the 7th Congress of the European Skull Base Society, Fulda, 2005.

Marangos N, Papadopoulou A, Papadopoulos A: Strategy in the Treatment of Bilateral Acoustic Neurinomas. Skull Base 16, 1055: 958616, Skull Base 17, Presentation at the 9th Congress of the European Skull Base Society, Prague, 2007..

Masterton RB: Role of the central auditory system in hearing: the new direction. Trends in Neuroscience, 15(8), 280-285, 1992.

Matthies C, Thomas S, Moshrefi M, Lesinski-Schiedat A, Frohne C, Battmer RD, Lenarz T, Samii M: Auditory brainstem implants: current neurosurgical experiences and perspective. J Laryngol Otol Suppl(27);32-6, 2000.

Mautner VF, Lindenau M et al: The neuroimaging and clinical spectrum of neurofibromatosis 2." Neurosurgery 38(5): 880-5; discussion 885-6, 1996.

McCreery DG, Yuen TGH, Agnew WF, and Bullara LA: A characterization of the effects on neuronal excitability resulting from prolonged microstimulation with chornically implanted microelectrodes, IEEE Trans. Biomed. Eng., 44, 831-939, 1997.

McCreery DB, Shannon RV, Moore JK, Chatterjee M: Acessing the tonotopic organization of the ventral cochlear nucleus by intranuclear microstimulation. IEEE Trans Rehabil Eng 6(4):391-9, 1998.

McCreery DB, Yuen T, Agnew WF, Bullara LA: Stimulation with chronically implanted microelectrodes in the cochlear nucleus of the cat: histologic and physiologic effects. Hear Res 62(1):42-56, 1993.

McCreery DB, Yuen TG, Agenew WF, Bullara LA: Stimulus parameters affecting tissue injury during microstimulation in the cochlear nucleus of the cat. Hear Res 15(77): 105-15, 1994.

McCreery DB, Yuen TG, Bullara LA: Chronic microstimulation in the feline ventral cochlear nucleus: physiologic and histologic effects. Hear Res 149(1-2):223-38, 2000.

McCreery D, Losinsky A, Pikov V, Liu X: Microelectrode array for chronic deep-brain microstimulation and recording . IEEE Trans Biomed Eng. 53(4):726-37, 2006.

McDermott HJ, McKay CM, Vandali AE: A new portable sound processor for the University of Melbourne/Nucleus Limited multielectrode cochlear implant. J Acoust Soc Am 91:3367-3371, 1992.

Mueller J, Behr R, Knaus C, Milewski C, Schoen F, Helms J: Electrical stimulation of the auditory pathway in deaf patients following acoustic neurinoma surgery and initial results with a new auditory brainstem implant system. Adv Otorhinolaryngol 57:229-902, 2001.

Mueller J: Die apparative Versorgung der Schwerhörigkeit: Cochlea- Implantate und Hirnstammimplantate- Aktuelle Entwicklungen der letzten 10 Jahre. Laryngo-Rhino- Otol 84 (1):60-69, 2005.

Nagafuchi M: Intelligibility of distorted speech sounds shifted in frequency and time in normal children, Audiology, 15, 326-337, 1976.

Nakatomi H, Kumakawa K, Usui M, Morita A, Kaga K, Seki Y, Komatsuzaki A: Multichannel Auditory Brainstem Implant in Japan: Factors Associated with Audiological Outcome. Skull Base 17; 1055: 981780, Skull Base 17, Presentation at the 9th Congress of the European Skull Base Society, Prague, 2007.

Nevison B, Laszig R, Sollmann WP, Lenarz T, Sterkers O, Ramsden R, Fraysse B, Manrique M, Rask-Andersen H, Garcia-Ibanez, Colletti V, van Wallenberg E: Results from a European clinical investigation of the Nucleus multichannel auditory brainstem implant. Ear Hear 23(3):170-83, 2002.

Nevison B: European ABI Experience and the Quality of Life Debate. Skull Base 17; 1055: 984022, Skull Base 17, Presentation at the 9th Congress of the European Skull Base Society, Prague, 2007..

Nilsson MJ, Soli SD, and Sullivan J: Development of a hearing in noise test for the measurement of speech reception threshold, J. Acoust. Soc. Am., 95, 1085-1099, 1994.

O´Driscoll M, Mawman D, Ramsden R: Intraoperative EABR and post-operative hearing in the ABI. Wiener Medizinische Wochenschrift 156 (119):45, 2006.

Otto SR, Shannon, R.V., Brackmann, D.E., Hitselberger, W.E., Staller, S., and Menapace, C: The multichannel auditory brainstem implant: Performance in 20 patients, Otolaryngology, Head and Neck Surgery, 118(3), 291-303, 1998.

Otto SR, Ebinger K, Staller SJ: Clinical trials with the auditory brainstem implant. In Cochlear Implants, Waltzmann S and Cohne N, eds., p 357-366. Thieme Medical Publishers Inc., New York, 2000.

Otto SR, Brackman DE, Hitselberger WE, Shannon R, Kuchta J: The Multichannel Auditory Brainstem Implant Update: Performance in 61 Patients. Journal of Neurosurgery, 2002.

Otto SR, Ebinger K, Staller S: Clinical trials with the auditory brainstem implant. Cochlear Implants Waltzman S and Cohen N, eds:357-366, 2000.

Otto SR, Shannon R, Brackmann D: The multichannel auditory brainstem implant (ABI): Results in 20 patients. Otolaryngol Head Neck Surg 118:291-303, 1998.

Otto SR, Staller S: Multichannel auditory brain stem implant: case studies comparing fitting strategies and results. Ann Otol Rhinol Laryngol Suppl 166:36-39, 1995.

Otto SR, Brackman DE, Hitselberger WE, Shannon RV: Brainstem electronic implants for bilateral anacusis following surgical removal of cerebello pontine angle lesions. Otolaryngol Clin North Am 34:485-499, 2001.

Otto SR, House WF, Brackmann DE, Hitselberger WE, Nelson RA: Auditory brain stem implant: effect of tumor size and preoperative hearing level on function. Ann Otol Rhinol Laryngol 99:789-790, 1990.

Otto SR, Shannon RV, Brackmann DE, Hitselberger WE, Staller S, Menapace C: The multichannel auditory brain stem implant: performance in twenty patients. Otolaryngol Head Neck Surg 118:291-303, 1998.

Otto SR, Waring MD, Kuchta J: Neural response telemetry and auditory/nonauditory sensations in 15 recipients of auditory brainstem implants. J Am Acad Audiol 16(4):219-27, 2005.

Parry DM, Eldridge R: Neurofibromatosis 2 (NF2): clinical characteristics of 63 affected individuals and clinical evidence for heterogeneity." Am J Med Genet 52(4): 450-61, 1994.

Pollack P, Gaio JM, Perret J: Parkinson´s disease and parkinsonian syndromes. Rev Prat 9:39(8):647-51, 1989.

Prochazka A, Mushahwar VK, McCreery DB: Neural prostheses. J Physiol 15(533):99-109, 2001.

Quester R, Schroder R: Topographic anatomy of the cochlear nuclear region at the floor of the fourh ventricle in humans. J Neurosurg 91(3):466-76, 1999.

Quester R, Schroder R, Klug N: Optimization of microsurgical operation technique to insert auditory brainstem implants: the results of a morphometric study. HNO 52(8): 706-13, 2004.

Rosen S: Temporal information in speech and its relevance for cochlear implants, in Philos. Trans. Royal Soc. London Ser. B Biol. Sci., 336, 367, 1992.

Rutherford SA, Thorne JA, King AT, Neef M, O´Driscoll M, Henderson L, Saeed SR, Ramsden RT: Auditory Brainstem Implantation in Children with Cochlear Nerve Aplasia/Dysplasia: Preliminary Report of Three Cases. Skull Base 17; 1055: 981741, Presentation at the 9th Congress of the European Skull Base Society, Prague, 2007.

Ruttledge MH, Phelan CM, et al: Type of Mutation in the NF2 Gene Frequently Determines Severity of Disease. Am J Hum Genet 59: 331-342, 1996.

Sainio M, Strachan T, et al: Presymptomatic DNA and MRI diagnosis of neurofibromatosis 2 with mild clinical course in an extended pedigree. Neurology 45(7): 1314-22, 1995.

Schlake HP, Goldbrunner RH, Milewski C, Krsuss J, Trautner H, Behr R, Sorensen N, Helms J, Roosen K: Intraoperative electromyographic monitoring of the lower cranial motor nerves (LCN IX-XII) in skull base surgery. Clin Neurol Neurosurg 103(2): 72-82, 2001.

Schlake HP, Goldbrunner R, Siebert M, Behr R, Roosen K: Intraoperative electromyographic monitoring of extra-ocular motor nerves (Nn.III, VI) in skull base surgery. Acta Neurochirur 143(3):251-61, 2001.

Schreiner CE, Langner G: Laminar fine structure of frequency organization in auditory midbrain. Nature 24;388(6640);383-6, 2000.

Seki Y, Samejima N, Kumakawa K, Komatsuzaki A: Subtonsillar placement of auditory brainstem implant. Acta neurochir Suppl 87:85-87, 2003.

Seligman P.M. McDermott H.J: Architecture of the Spectra-22 speech processor. Annals of Otology, Rhinology and Laryngology, 104, Suppl. 166, 139-141, 1995.

Shannon RV, Fayad J, Moore J, Lo WM, Otto S, Nelson RA, O'Leary M: Auditory brainstem implant: II. Postsurgical issues and performance. Otolaryngology Head Neck Surg 108:634-642, 1993.

Shannon RV, Zenner HP, Wygonski J, Kamath V, Ekelid M: Speech recognition with primarily temporary cues. Science 270:303-304, 1995.

Shannon RV: Multichannel electrical stimulation of the auditory nerve in man. I. Basic psychophysics. Hear Res 11:157-189, 1983.

Shannon RV: Multichannel electrical stimulation of the auditory nerve in man. II. Channel interaction. Hear Res 12:1-16, 1983.

Shannon RV: Quantitative comparison of electrically and acoustically evoked auditory perception: implications for the location of perceptual mechanisms. Prog Brain Res 97:261-269, 1993.

Shannon RV, Fayad J, Moore J, Lo WW, Otto S, Nelson RA, O'Leary M: Auditory brainstem implant: II. Postsurgical issues and performance. Otolaryngol Head Neck Surg 108:634-642, 1993.

Shannon, RV: Multichannel electrical stimulation of the auditory nerve in man: II Channel interaction. Hearing Research, 12, 1-16, 1983.

Shannon, RV: Loudness summation as a measure of channel interaction in a multichannel cochlear implant. In Cochlear Implants, R.A. Schindler and M.M. Merzenich, Eds., Raven Press, New York, 1985.

Shannon, RV., Zeng FG, and Wygonski J: Speech recognition using only temporal cues, in The Auditory Processing of Speech: From Sounds to Words, M.E.H. Schouten (Ed.), Mouton-DeGruyter, New York, pp 263-274, 1992.

Shannon RV, Fayad J, Moore JK, Lo W, O'Leary M, Otto S and Nelson RA: Auditory brainstem implant. II: Post-surgical issues and performance, Otolaryngology, Head and Neck Surgery, 108, 635-643, 1993.

Shannon RV, Zeng F.-G, Wygonski, J, Kamath V, and Ekelid M: Speech recognition with primarily temporal cues, Science, 270, 303-304, 1995.

Shannon RV, Moore J, McCreery D, and Portillo F: Threshold-distance measures from electrical stimulation of human brainstem, IEEE Trans. on Rehabilitation Engineering, 5, 1-5, 1997.

Shannon RV, Zeng FG, and Wygonski J: Speech recognition with altered spectral distribution of envelope cues, J. Acoust. Soc. Amer., 104, 1998.

Shannon RV, Carner M, Colletti L, Colletti V: Comparison of ABI results in NF2 and non-tumor patients. Wiener Medizinische Wochenschrift 156 (119):45-46, 2006.

Skrivan J, Zverina E, Kluh J, Betka J, Tichy T, Kraus J: Our Experience with Auditory Brainstem Implants. Skull Base 17, 1055, 984019, Presentation at the 9th Congress of the European Skull Base Society, Prague, 2007.

Sollmann WP, Laszig R: Anatomical Findings and Surgical Experiences in 92 Cases Using the Nucleus Multichannel Auditory Brainstem Implant. Skull Base 15; 1055: 916404, Skull Base 17, Presentation at the 7th Congress of the European Skull Base Society, Fulda, 2005.

Sterkers O, Buzorg-Grayeli A, Ambert-Dahan E, Bomccara D, Kalamarides M, Sollmann WP, Rey A: Auditory brainstem implant in NF2 and other otologic indications. Wiener Medizinische Wochenschrift 156 (119):44, 2006.

Sturm V, Kuhner A, Schmitt HP, Assmus H, Stock G: Chronic electrical stimulation of the thalamic unspecific activating system in a patient with coma due to midbrain and upper brain stem infarction. Acta Neurochir 47(3-4):235-44, 1979.

Stypulkowski PH, van den Honert C: Physiological properties of the electrically stimulated auditory nerve. I. Compound action potential recordings. Hear Res 14:205-223, 1984.

Terr LI, Mobley JP, House WF: Biocompatibility of the central electroauditory prosthesis and the human cochlear nuclei. Om J Otol 10(5):339-42, 1989.

Tiffany WR, Bennett DA: Intelligibility of slow-played speech, J. Speech Hearing Res., 4, 248-258, 1961.

Trabalzini F, Scienzia R, Pavesi G: Digisonic SP Auditory Brainstem Implant in NF2 Patients. Skull Base 17, Presentation at the 9th Congress of the European Skull Base Society, Prague, 2007.

Van Tasell DJ, Soli SD, Kirby VM, and Widin GP: Speech waveform envelope cues for consonant recognition, J. Acoust. Soc. Amer., 82, 1152-1161, 1987.

Vercueil L, Pollak P, Fraix V, Caputo E, Moro E, Benazzouz A, Xie J, Koudsie A, Benabid AL: Deep brain stimulation in the treatment of severe dystonia. J Neurol 248(8): 695-700, 2001.

Vercueil L, Krack P, Pollak P: Results of deep brain stimulation for dystonia: a critical reappraisal. Mov Disorders 17 supp 3:89-93, Review, 2002.

Voges J, Schroder R, Treuer H, Pastyr O, Schlegel W, Lorenz WJ, Sturm V: CT-guided and computer assisted stereotactic biopsy. Technique, results, indications. Acta Neurochir 125(1-4):142-9, 1993.

Voges J, Waerzeggers Y, Maarouf M, Lehrke R, Koulousakis A, Lenartz D, Sturm V: Deep Brain Stimulation: Long-term analysis of complications caused by hardware and surgery- a single center experience. J Neurol Neurosurg Psychiatry 30:1-9, 2006.

Waring MD: Electrically evoked auditory brainstem response monitoring of auditory brainstem implant integrity during facial nerve tumor surgery. Laryngoscope 102:1293-1295, 1992.

Waring MD: Auditory brain-stem responses evoked by electrical stimulation of the cochlear nucleus in human subjects. Electroencephalogr Clin Neurophysiol 96:338-347, 1995.

Waring MD: Intraoperative electrophysiologic monitoring to assist placement of auditory brain stem implant. Ann Otol Rhinol Laryngol Suppl 166:33-36, 1995.

Waring MD: Properties of auditory brainstem responses evoked by intra-operative electrical stimulation of the cochlear nucleus in human subjects. Electroencephalogr Clin Neurophysiol 100:538-548, 1996.

Waring MD: Refractory properties of auditory brain-stem responses evoked by electrical stimulation of human cochlear nucleus: evidence of neural generators. Electroencephalogr Clin Neurophysiol 108:331-344, 1998.

Waring MD, Ponton CW, Don M: Activating separate ascending auditory pathways Aproduces different human thalamic/cortical responses. Hear Res 130:219-229, 1999a

Welling DB, Guida M, et al: Mutational spectrum in the neurofibromatosis type 2 gene in sporadic and familial schwannomas." Hum Genet 98(2): 189-93, 1996.

Wishart JH: Case of tumors of the skull, dura mater and brain." Edinburgh Med Surg J 18: 393-397, 1822

Yamamoto T, Katayama Y, Oshima H, Fukaya C, Kawamata T, Tsbokawa T: Deep brain stimulation therapy for a persistent vegetative state. Acta Neurochiru Suppl 79_79-82, 2002.

Zverina E, Betka J, Skrivan J, Kraus J, Kluh J, Belsan T: Vestibular Schwannoma: Microsurgery after Partial Removal and Stereoradiosurgery. Skull Base 15, Presentation at the 7th Congress of the European Skull Base Society, Fulda, 2005.

Zwolan TA, Collins LM, and Wakefield GH: Electrode discrimination and speech recognition in postlingually deafened adult cochlear implant subjects, J. Acoust. Soc. Amer., 102(6), 3673-3685, 1997.

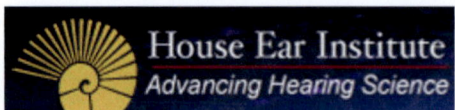

House Ear Institute
Advancing Hearing Science

April 4th, 2001

Johannes Kuchta, M.D.
Department of Auditory Implants and Perception
House Ear Institute, 2100 W. 3rd Street
Los Angeles, CA 90057
mail: jkuchta@hei.org

To: Multichannel ABI (ABI24) Recipients
Re: Special MRI´s of ABI electrode array area

We are studying the relationship between the exact position of your ABI electrode
array and your responses to it.
This information will be helpful in fitting and implanting ABI´s.
We are continuing a previous study of this type and would greatly appreciate your
help, since you are among the few individuals who can answer the questions we
are posing.
Therefore, we would like to ask that you have a special MRI done of your ABI
electrode array region as soon as possible. Below please find the protocol which
should be used to help properly identify the location of the array.
Please let us know if you have already had such a post-operative MRI study
performed elsewhere, or let us know when you have scheduled this test.
Please have your radiologist make a copy of the scans and send them to us:
If you need help obtaining insurance coverage for this test or any other assistance
please let me know and I will try to provide a prescription.

Guidelines for MRI evaluation (W Lo/V Waluch-St Vincent Medical Center)
Basic sequences through posterior cranial fossa, e.g.,
transverse T1-weightened (TR 580/TE 15/ 2 Acq) 3-mm thick
transverse Gd-T1 WI (580/15/2) 3-mm
transverse T2-WI (5700/90/8 ET) 3-mm

Optional additional sequences, e.g.,
transverse fat-suppressed Gd-T1 WI
Coronal Gd-T1 WI
Sagittal Gd-T1 WI
To increase conspicuity of electrodes, use gradient-echo sequence

Sincerely,

Johannes Kuchta

Categories of ABI position
for postoperative MRI- image classification

(defined in collaboration with Jane Moore, Anatomical Dep. HEI, 2001)

      A) deep in recess, in 4th ventricle
      B) over CN at taenia
      C) half out of recess
      D) outside the recess

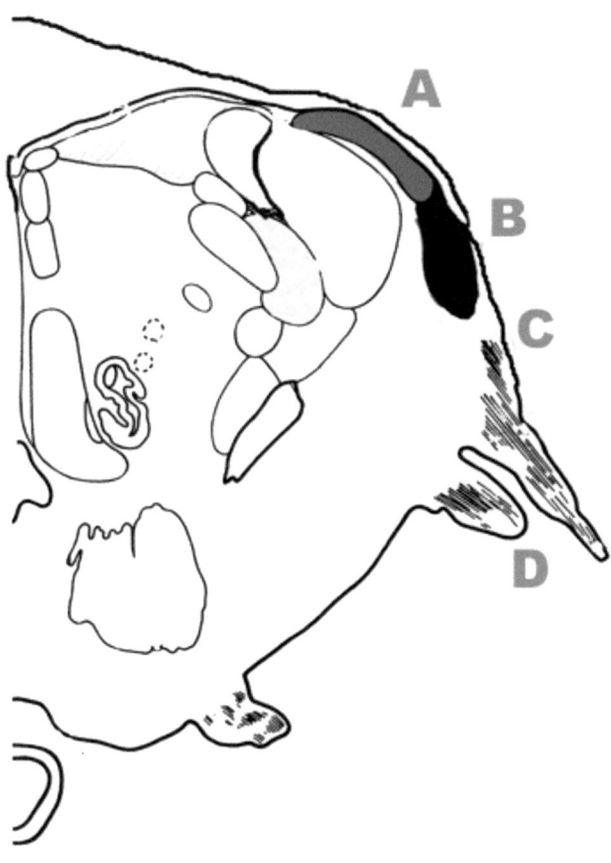

abi mult otto alle nov01.html — 30.03.2006 20:06 Uhr

M/C ABI	Implant Date	Test Date	MTS WORD%	MTS STRESS%	SERT%	NU-CHIPS%	CID SENTS (S)%	CONS (S)%	CONS (V)%	CONS (SV)%	VOWELS (S)%	VOWELS (V)%	VOWELS (SV)%	CUNY SENTS (S)%	CUNY SENTS (V)%	CUNY SENTS (SV)%
1	28.09.92	18.12.92	21	79	45			13	30	49	12	50	58	0	15	37
1	28.09.92	16.02.93						21	36	63	29	50	71	2	28	40
1		18.03.93	21	67	30			13	40	43	29	58	75	3	33	48
1		20.10.93	27	60	70			24	38	56	21	54	92	1	26	55
1		15.06.94	63	96	60			28	39	55	29	33	71	3	21	58
1		30.11.94	50	92	57	70	0	19	34	56	42	46	79	5	26	65
1		11.07.95	71	92	53	65	0	33	35	65	38	62	79	6	35	57
1		19.08.96	46	96	57	72	6	30	35	61	29	75	71	5	12	49
1		12.11.97	63	96	70	48	10	34	38	70	54	67	83	2	29	69
1	28.09.92	10.11.99	58	88	67	68	24	39	13	69	67	79	83	8	23	75
1		20.11.00	88	100	80	57	20	37			54		83	5		60
2	07.12.92	02.02.93	25	92				18	40	63	12	62	83	0	32	67
2		13.05.93	67	92	35			33	33	61	12	75	83	2	46	66
2		22.02.94	52	95	50			16	43	43	21	62	88	0	43	50
2		07.03.95	27	87	50	32		19	45	50	12	67	83	0	64	83
2		15.02.96	71	96	57	42	2	21	38	53	29	71	79	1	51	73
2		19.02.97	33	83	50	46	0	28	33	53	29	79	71	0	59	66
2		28.05.99	29	67	50											
3	11.01.93	22.02.93						26	49	68	33	83	92	0	54	81
3		25.02.93	30	79	65											
3		05.04.93	38	67	70			34		71	33		83	0		87
3		06.04.93						33		84	29		92	1	0	81
3		12.08.93	25	79	55			25	46	88	33	79	79	1	58	96
3		04.11.93	50	75	50			30	55	71	17	92	83	6	52	91
3		02.06.94	46	92	47			25	55	69	21	67	88	1	66	85
3		03.01.95	50	92	57	54	0	18	34	67	17	75	83	1	61	92
3		23.10.95	71	88	77	71	2	31	40	81	38	75	88	0	45	86
3		23.04.97	46	79	72	56	0	20	52	69	29	75	83	0	62	79
4	22.05.93	27.07.93	13	75	45			21	39	53	29	67	83	4	40	64
4		21.10.93						19	36	79	12	46	92	5	55	82
4		20.06.94	46	67	43			25	40	83	29	42	75	4	53	73
4		22.02.95	42	88	57	74	0	23	35	86	38	54	75	2	66	85
4		15.10.96	33	88	43	56	0	28	38	79	17	75	83	1	42	79
4		03.06.98	33	75	41	46	0	0	0	0	0	0	0	0	0	0
4		19.05.99	21	75	57	60	0	24	46	65	17	83	75	1	52	86
4		13.12.00	17	75	62	41		20	48	59	25	71	75	0	68	76
5	01.11.93	08.12.93	8	42	40			0	30	25	29	67	62	0	0	18
5		07.03.94	46	83	40			20	23	34	25	62	67	3	5	24
5		07.06.94	50	79	63			16	28	49	38	54	67	3	6	24
5		13.09.94	46	88	60	70	0	23	29	40	33	58	62	0	5	29
5		11.01.95	63	83	47	67	14	20	30	36	25	62	75	7	3	34
5		10.05.95	54	88	60	61	2	23	41	43	33	67	71	0	7	37
5		11.10.95	46	88	77	60	0	26	36	49	33	50	75	9	11	46
5		12.11.96	79	96	87	76	14	28	48	59	67	71	88	22	16	65
5		10.12.97	88	96	80	76	46	20	23	49	67	42	79	24	0	30
5		08.05.00	88	96	67	0	28	37	0	0	79	0	0	15	0	0
5		08.05.01			80		28							5		

abi mult otto alle nov01.html   30.03.2006 20:06 Uhr

6	19.11.93	07.04.94	9	50	25			15	38	30	0	42	33	7	13	33
6		26.07.94	33	92	20	24		8	33	41	8	75	71			
6		19.08.94	21	79										2	25	43
6		25.04.95	29	79	37	30	0	6	34	36	21	71	54	4	25	47
6		31.07.96	42	83	43	36	0	14	39	29	17	58	67	0	19	18
6	19.11.93	16.07.97	0	0	40	0	0	13	40	46	21	62	54	0	0	23
6		17.07.98	17	75	47	38	0	8		52	8		62			
7	07.04.94	28.06.94	30	71	30				21	50				0	11	28
7		03.10.94	30	67	37	42	0	18	29	48	38	62	67	0	28	69
7		13.02.95	38	71	50	37	0	16	38	40	42	62	71	2	23	75
7		05.06.95	46	71	43	54	0	33	36	46	46	54	79	0	17	51
8	08.07.94		0	0	0	0	0	0	0	0	0	0	0	0	0	0
9	26.07.94	01.09.94	38	88	70	54	0	10	26	40	17	79	58	2	48	82
9		08.12.94	50	96	70	60	0	40	34	76	46	71	79	24	54	95
9		12.04.95	71	96	70	76	45	53	39	78	54	75	79	25	67	95
9		20.07.95	75	100	70	80	50	66	49	90	50	75	86	55	66	97
9		16.10.95	83	96	73	86	44	58	40	83	71	71	83	49	38	96
9		17.10.96	71	88	80	74	70	60	48	90	62	67	88	65	42	100
9		16.10.97	88	100	80	86	54	66	40	95	62	75	88	66	58	100
9		08.10.98	63	88	70	84	62	63	30	89	62	67	88	53	63	98
9		07.10.99	79	96	87	82	46	57	40	89	50	92	92	64	55	97
9		05.10.00						52		88	62		100	51		97
9		04.10.01	88	100	97	88		70		91	54		96			
10	28.07.94	08.09.94	58	83	50	58	0	33	30	45	17	33	71	1	2	13
10		15.12.94	71	88	67	72	2	10	25	63	29	58	71	7	7	25
10		15.03.95	75	96	83	72	0	45	28	75	42	58	71	14	8	31
10		13.07.95	83	96	83	70	12	41	30	80	46	50	75	21	9	38
10		19.10.95	88	100	83	70	12	38	40	78	42	67	50	14	4	37
10		16.09.96	79	92	83	82	8	54	31	83	33	67	75	14	8	43
10		07.10.97	83	96	83	83	26	59	39	76	29	67	67	11	11	36
10		06.10.98	88	96	87	92	10	56	43	86	29	62	67	17	5	35
10		13.09.99	92	100	90	86	10	58	39	81	54	54	88	21	3	54
10		26.07.00	88	96	100	86	28	65	38	90	46	62	71	19	9	48
10		25.07.01	79	96	100	86		58			62		79			
11	19.08.94	12.10.94	29	71	50	32	0	16	46	56	21	50	46	1	17	41
11		01.02.95	42	88	77	49	0	26	35	54	33	46	71	2	17	65
11		17.05.95	67	92	67	54	12	48	56	61	50	54	62	17	28	85
11		05.10.95	83	100	70	84	6	49	39	88	50	54	83	35	22	87
11		08.02.96	83	100	80	66	18	40	40	83	46	58	67	55	24	92
11		13.02.97	92	100	93	76	22	53	45	75	50	71	96	40	31	93
11		05.03.98	92	96	87	74	16	59	39	91	29	50	92	41	22	93
11		04.03.99	63	96	93	79	6	53	44	88	42	71	88	30	36	88
11		08.12.99	96	100	90	72	40	48	36	90	58	50	83	31	30	91
11		10.11.00	100	100	93	84	30	53	48	89	50	50	88	36		90
12	11.10.94	28.11.94	17	75	37	32	0	20	43	49	25	62	92	0	55	83
12		02.03.95	25	79	53	68	0	18	46	66	33	58	71	1	72	90
12		14.09.95	54	88	63	56	2	21	28	66	33	62	79	4	55	98
12		22.02.96	46	83	47	76	4	20	49	61	38	58	83	5	52	91
12		25.03.97	63	88	60	73	4	58	44	83	46	62	75	19	51	98
12		24.09.98	63	88	0	0	0	0	0	0	0	0	0	0	0	0

abi mult otto alle nov01.html   30.03.2006 20:06 Uhr

12		10.03.99	75	96	77	86	24	38	46	84	46	71	71	18	48	99
12		21.11.00	79	100	83	74	0	38		86	38		71	24		94
13	10.11.94	08.03.95	38	67	30	48	0	26	38	48	8	58	79	1	19	32
13		28.06.95	75	83	73	60	2	24	40	63	50	75	83	0	14	63
13		27.09.95	88	92	80	78	50	54	31	81	67	88	92	64	19	93
13		03.01.96	92	96	87	90	64	56	36	94	62	71	96	61	23	98
13		01.05.96	96	96	83	84	50	65	44	95	67	75	92	58	24	97
13		25.11.96	96	96	90	90	52	68	39	94	50	88	92	53	17	94
13		10.07.97	88	100	80	84	16	50	41	91	50	79	71	13	10	85
13		09.04.98	92	96	90	82	44	63	30	91	62	75	92	43	14	97
13		08.04.99	92	96	87	92	30	59	40	81	42	40	96	36	34	91
13		10.04.00	100	100	97	86	46	56	38	96	672	83	96	42	26	92
13		16.04.01	96	100		82		53			46			42		
14	10.01.95	23.03.95	8	71	47	40	0	10	38	34	21	58	71	1	40	66
14		25.07.95	13	50	40	44	0	6	36	40	8	58	75	3	64	83
15	24.01.95	28.03.95	29	79	30	38	0	10	19	28	33	42	67	0	10	23
15		27.07.95	33	83	57	29	0	9	26	28	25	42	62	7	21	47
15		26.10.95	38	88	60	42	2	14	33	39	29	71	67	3	17	45
15		31.01.96	58	92	73	62	0	21	34	54	21	79	75	6	14	40
15		14.05.96	46	88	70	60	2	18	24	51	29	50	79	0	11	42
15		09.04.97	42	75	77	48	0	14	31	36	25	67	75	0	10	26
15		09.07.98	38	67	55	52	0	11	42	40	42	54	88	0	6	22
15		15.07.99	33	75	57	48	0	20	35	45	25	58	96	5	10	34
15		18.09.00	54	92	60	52	6	27	34	48	58	62	62	0	6	48
15		10.09.01	71	92	70	42		21	30	55	29	71	71	8	13	47
16	31.01.95	04.04.95	33	87	53	44	0	9	33	58	25	83	83	0	62	92
16		09.08.95	46	88	47	0	54	18	41	79	21	75	96	7	84	94
16		16.07.96	29	75	70	54	0	20	43	65	42	75	100	0	78	88
16		21.10.98	25	75	63	62	0	20	35	61	21	83	83	0	75	93
16		05.05.00	13	88	66	47	0	18	51	68	21	79	79	0	48	76
17	10.03.95	04.05.95	21	88	57	38	0	19	33	48	10	58	67	0	49	60
17		31.08.95	50	92	67	62	0	21	43	56	25	71	88	0	52	88
17		27.11.95	50	92	73	56	2	23	46	63	38	71	88	2	44	90
17		11.03.96	42	92	77	54	0	36	46	84	38	54	88	4	48	77
17		20.06.96	54	92	77	62	2	29	54	78	33	62	83	6	54	100
17	10.03.95	05.09.97	75	92	79	56	0	35	49	80	33	67	92	1	53	99
17		12.04.99	92	100	77	76	4	48	45	84	42	67	83	9	43	94
18	09.06.95	02.08.95	29	71	50	40	0	5	36	34	33	50	62	0	11	7
18		06.11.95	30	54	57	36	0	10	26	39	33	54	54	0	12	12
18		20.02.96	21	58	60	52	0	8	33	45	25	54	54	0	13	25
18		29.05.96	25	75	60	55	0	10	33	43	25	54	71	1	18	27
18		21.08.96	29	88	60	48	0	14	21	48	21	54	79	1	15	33
18		06.05.97	50	79	70	62	2	14	16	48	33	58	67	0	9	30
18		11.05.98	46	88	57	52	0	13	31	56	42	46	62	1	11	40
18		01.04.99	46	88	50	52	0	13	35	48	33	50	75	0	0	39
18		20.04.00	46	92	63	63	0	15	31	41	29	38	75	3	12	53
18		03.05.01	50	92	63	40		13	24	41	29	54	75			
19	06.11.95	10.01.96	28	83	30	30	0	10	37	38	4	71	71	0	23	20
19		03.04.96	58	88	53	46	2	9	44	49	21	67	88	1	23	40
19		05.06.96	38	75	73	52	0	20	35	51	17	83	79	0	40	52

abi mult otto alle nov01.html

19		12.12.96	25	79	40	42	0	15	45	56	25	79	79	0	22	26
19		18.09.98	29	83	38	42	0	11	45	61	21	83	88	0	34	30
20	14.11.95	18.01.96	21	75	50	36	0	11	40	54	21	54	83	1	23	25
20		22.04.96	25	71	47	26		15	43	51	25	58	67	1	23	42
20		23.07.96	21	83	60	53	0	21	50	59	25	54	58	1	45	45
20		24.10.96	21	88	63	48	0	16	43	64	38	79	71	3	36	55
20		07.01.97	25	92	67	56	2	21	54	69	46	67	75	4	22	59
20		08.01.98	21	88	60	32	0	18	45	70	21	67	79	2	40	51
20		14.01.99	13	71	73	34	0	15	43	61	38	62	92	3	36	51
20		13.01.00	38	83	63	46	0	14	38	69	46	75	79	2	35	55
20		10.01.01	63	92	90	58		17	33	67	42	54	75	6	27	65
21	08.12.95	06.02.96	33	67	46	42	0	9	15	26	29	54	50	0	28	41
21		23.05.96	25	88	63	38	0	9	28	33	25	67	75	0	23	69
21		05.09.96	29	83	60	38	0	8	45	54	29	54	62	0	26	53
21		25.03.99	42	83	60	48	0	23	41	54	33	54	75	2	24	65
22	23.01.96		0	0	0	0	0	0	0	0	0	0	0	0	0	0
23	26.03.96		0	0	0	0	0	0	0	0	0	0	0	0	0	0
24	17.05.96		0	0	0	0	0	0	0	0	0	0	0	0	0	0
25	28.05.96	26.07.96	13	75	43	46	0									
25		31.10.96	9	73	47	34	17	14	31	34	17	58	71	3	6	18
25		20.03.97	17	58	60	38	0	18	23	29	33	54	67	0	6	15
25		31.10.97	38	79	41	63	0	19	38	46	29	46	67	0	2	18
25		22.09.98	38	83	62	42	0	13	30	49	46	38	54	0	11	46
26	07.06.96	29.10.96	8	58	47	27	0	17	67	75	19	38	46	0	11	33
26		11.02.97	21	83	53	36	0	11	40	44	21	62	67	0	15	25
26		28.07.97	25	75	55	36	0	17	30	46	29	58	58	0	20	31
27	25.06.96	08.08.96	42	83	53	38	0	8	50	58	46	83	75	0	81	76
27		15.11.96	46	83	50	68	0	21	51	61	54	75	83	1	66	79
27		06.03.97	42	83	83	44	4	18	39	64	33	71	83	6	79	91
27		08.08.97	38	92	60	0	0	0	0	0	0	0	0	0	0	0
27		23.04.98	50	71	70	43	2	24	58	73	42	92	88	0	60	89
27		27.04.00	50	88	63	46	0	22	42	69	33	88	92	4	74	96
27		22.03.01	54	88		63		22	40	73	33		88	2		88
28	12.07.96	08.10.96	58	100	63	54	0	16	30	48	12	30	50	0	23	62
28		20.01.97	58	88	60	52	0	25	40	70	50	75	79	1	23	66
28		21.04.97	50	92	79	69	8	29	40	68	42	62	75	8	21	85
28		03.12.98	54	83	80	56	0	23	48	63	46	83	67	0	33	73
29	25.10.96	06.12.96	4	42	37	42	0	5	33	30	12	46	46	0	20	19
29		13.03.97	25	54	33	39	0	6	25	29	21	46	42	0	11	17
29		19.06.97	13	71	38	38	0	5	39	35	12	58	54	0	9	20
29		02.10.97	21	63	38	24	0	8	25	40	17	75	83	0	10	19
29		29.01.98	29	75	38	46	0	10	30	34	12	62	58	0	14	23
29		28.01.99	21	58	38	34	0	12	33	48	8	71	67	0	8	26
29		28.01.00	38	83	37	20	0	10	31	48	12	58	67	0	18	25
29		07.02.01	25	75	50	44		8		39	42		58			
30	19.11.96	14.01.97	13	63	53	38	0	15	36	44	25	58	58	1	19	31
30		16.04.97	13	50	33	36	0	18	43	51	50	75	79	0	24	44
30		24.07.97	33	67	33	48	0	24	39	49	25	79	79	0	37	37
30		14.11.97	29	63	60	34	0	22	45	43	33	71	83	0	28	52
30		08.09.98	25	71	60	44	0	15	44	59	38	58	75	0	24	58

30		11.08.99	58	96	60	56	0	23	41	63	46	62	75	0	41	55
30		09.08.00	63	88	43	62	0	27	32	60	38	62	88	3	37	56
30		08.08.01	50	83	67	38		20		57	62		71	0	34	71
31	28.01.97	19.03.97	17	79	73	42	0	17	38	44	25	58	75	2	29	76
31		23.06.97	29	75	59	42	0	6	29	44	17	67	83	0	25	63
31		09.10.97	33	75	63	44	0	33	45	55	50	71	79	0	48	63
31		26.01.98	33	79	55	56	0	31	49	74	46	58	79	3	24	79
31		29.04.98	21	79	60	58	0	22	49	59	38	67	96	0	31	69
31		14.04.99	38	75	69	48	0	22	50	58	21	62	83	0	21	63
31		05.04.00	38	83	55	28	0	14	52	57	21	50	79	0	33	56
32	12.02.97	08.04.97	8	42	43	28	0	13	40	41	12	54	62	0	40	41
32		14.07.97	33	75	60	46	0	15	36	45	25	58	75	0	43	39
32		20.10.97	29	83	50	48	0	14	40	44	29	62	71	0	32	45
32		27.04.98	17	50	37	46	0	8	38	49	21	71	71	0	45	66
33	28.03.97	20.05.97	54	83	57	48	14	23	35	54	21	67	75	6	30	74
33	28.03.97	08.09.97	46	83	70	64	0	20	40	58	25	58	71	1	40	80
33		09.12.97	83	96	66	56	0	25	34	63	42	62	88	7	33	90
33		24.06.98	54	96	53	46	0	20	41	59	42	41	79	1	46	72
33		22.07.99	58	92	60	41	0	19	41	58	33	79	88	3	31	75
34	11.04.97	27.08.97	29	50	36	26	0	8	38	58	42	75	71	0	45	37
34		17.11.97	25	63	48	36	0	11	30	44	29	58	79	1	59	58
34		09.03.98	71	88	62	72	2	39	50	78	42	75	79	0	54	77
34		15.07.98	63	92	47	64	2	25	39	56	33	62	88	4	51	73
34		12.07.99	83	96	67	68	0	21	34	61	46	62	80	2	50	75
34		24.07.00	71	88	72	70	4	24	45	72	46	58	79	0	51	66
34		08.10.01	75	92	66	70		25	33	60	38	46	75	2	47	80
35	22.04.97	12.06.97	46	67	72	37	0	10	26	40	8	42	38	0	8	39
35		22.09.97	42	79	76	32	0	7	46	40	25	38	38	0	13	52
35		04.05.98	38	88	60	34	0	11	34	58	12	50	67	1	22	64
35		24.08.98	50	92	63	42		16	40	68	21	58	62	0	29	67
35		10.05.99	63	96	67	36	0	20	29	63	21	50	50	0	22	58
35		22.06.00	38	92	67	44	0	19	36	68	21	54	62	0	34	68
35		30.07.01	54	92	79	24		16	23	55	42	42	71			
37	29.07.97	11.09.97	29	75	60	33	0	10	53	54	25	88	88	1	40	75
37		05.12.97	13	67	57	40	0	10	48	58	21	71	71	4	61	82
37		12.03.98	25	67	60	26	0	26	65	74	29	62	96	3	48	63
37		02.06.98	42	88	57	46	2	28	53	76	21	79	92	1	65	76
37		26.10.98	46	92	63	40	4	20	55	76	62	78	96	9	62	86
37		06.08.99	21	83	59	30	0	11	43	63	21	88	88	4	68	89
37		07.08.00	38	88	53	43	4	19	50	64	17	75	100	3	48	72
38	12.08.97	25.09.97	25	63	33	34	0	5	26	33	17	17	17	0	0	0
38		15.12.97	29	67	62	34	0	9	29	30	4	46	42	1	22	52
38		13.04.98	25	71	47	34	0	7	25	36	32	38	32	0	24	50
38		07.07.98	21	83	50	52	0	12	26	36	17	33	50	0	20	39
38		10.02.00	33	79	67	58	0	4	22	31	21	33	46	0	28	47
39	12.09.97	22.10.97	29	63	34	31	0	15	42	46	33	75	71	0	46	71
39		05.02.98	38	75	37	36	0	16	45	49	29	92	88	0	52	77
39		14.05.98	17	58	59	44	0	10	40	49	29	92	79	2	56	58
39		19.10.98	17	71	52	34	0	13	63	55	12	67	83	0	54	64
39		14.10.99	42	63	50	40	0	24	58	55	25	92	88	0	53	60

abi mult otto alle nov01.html   30.03.2006 20:06 Uhr

39		19.09.01	71	92	67	72		31		67	42			92	5	57	99
40	12.12.97	17.03.98	16	58	40	38	0	3	33	28	25	58	50			
40		15.06.99	21	50	47	26	0	14	30	41	25	62	62			
40		22.09.00	21	71	47											
41		10.10.01	42	83	70	44		25	38	71	31	39	54	0	5	15
42	16.01.98	19.02.98	21	79	60	26								0	17	47
42		18.05.98	63	100	73	34	0	18	25	46	8	75	88	4	33	60
42		30.10.98	42	83	83	42	0	25	38	61	21	71	75	5	26	60
42		01.03.99	42	79	83	66	0	26	33	55	25	54	79	5	36	61
42		06.03.00	33	83	78	46	0	18	36	55	29	58	83	2	36	67
44	20.02.98	24.03.98	8	50	59	42	0	11	58	43	21	79	92	3	44	46
44		06.08.98	29	63	50	44	0	12	40	55	29	67	96	0	44	65
44		12.11.98	50	100	70	64	4	25	44	61	46	58	96	12	35	83
44		18.02.99	63	88	80	72	6	46	43	65	62	79	100	7	52	78
44		03.06.99	79	96	70	78	0	30	41	60	46	75	79	13	45	94
44		01.06.00	75	96	77	60	10	36	38	68	62	67	92	7	53	87
44		08.06.01	83	100	77	76		47	29	71	58	67	88	27	59	91
45	24.03.98	27.05.98	17	67	47	44	0	8	39	49	8	62	67	7	20	50
45		23.11.98	42	96	70	52	2	17	34	45	12	67	62	10	32	51
45		02.05.99	25	75	67	62		24	33	49	17	58	62	7	31	60
45		26.10.00	33	75	63	60		15	37	63						
46	30.06.98	29.10.98	8	50	50	36	0	7	31	31	33	62	50	0	2	8
46		26.01.99	33	75	60	52	0	5	48	44	25	62	67	2	20	23
46		13.05.99	8	58	53	31	0	21	40	46	17	38	50	5	9	25
46		11.05.00	17	67	60	46	2	20	46	50	38	58	71	6	12	42
46		10.05.01	46	79	60	44		14	27	48	46	54	83	8		43
47	14.07.98	27.08.98	21	67	52	26	0	5	34	35	29	42	46	1	31	46
47		16.11.98	17	46	40	43	0	5	36	41	17	42	62	0	24	28
47		16.02.99	46	71	69	41	0	24	39	58	29	71	75	0	39	56
47		24.05.99	50	83	57	50	0	16	36	49	29	79	79	0	27	62
47		20.09.99	63	79	57	50	0	14	36	56	42	71	92	0	39	71
47		14.08.00	33	83	60	58	0	22	34	52	42	62	67	0	22	86
47		31.07.01	46	88	70	58		8	0	56	21		79			
48		25.02.99	29	88	53	42	0	0	0	0	30	0	50	0	0	0
48		11.06.99	38	83	63											
49	29.07.98	15.12.98	13	75	52	44	0	11	41	33	21	33	29	0	8	26
50	29.07.98	11.12.98	29	67	45	36	0	8	24	31	12	58	50	0	16	28
50		17.05.99	13	71	80	36	0	8	34	31	17	62	54	0	4	30
50		09.01.01	54	83	70	30		10	32	38	30	58	79	1	21	49
51	06.08.98	15.09.98	8	29	31	32	0	11	19	30	12	62	71			
51		07.12.98	8	67	43	20	0	9	36	35	8	46	46	0	4	7
51		08.03.99	33	67	27	36	0	9	31	43	25	62	75	0	6	13
51		17.06.99	25	79	34	36	0	2	44	41	21	54	75	0	5	12
51		12.06.00	38	75	37	35	0	4	36	29	12	46	62	2	4	23
51		11.06.01	42	67	40	44		3	12	38	12	62	71			
53	18.09.98	10.11.98	17	50	27	34	0	8	24	41	25	58	67	0	49	61
53		10.02.99	33	83	57	36	0	21	49	58	12	83	79	0	52	79
53		19.05.99	25	79	38	46	0	14	51	66	38	79	83	0	53	64
53		21.10.99	21	71	47	41	0	17	40	53	17	67	62	0	56	75
53		27.06.00	50	83	57	50	0	23	39	48	12	71	67	0	48	63

abi mult otto alle nov01.html   30.03.2006 20:06 Uhr

53		07.06.01	42	79	43	48		10	41	57	17	71	79	1	41	72
54	20.11.98	19.01.99	71	96	60	63	0	31	40	60	42	54	58	8	18	62
54		19.04.99	46	88	86	65	4	30	39	55	29	54	88	1	26	64
54		01.11.99	67	88	80	58	14	31	35	61	38	62	96	12	32	81
54		06.11.00	50	96	77	50	0	30	28	65	42	58	80	11	35	72
55	11.12.98	16.08.99	21	75	37	42	0	3	44	38	8	71	46	0	16	21
55		29.11.99	29	58	50	38	0	8	39	39	8	54	67	4	21	24
55		07.02.00	17	71	50	40	0	8	39	32	12	62	54	0	19	23
57	24.02.99	22.04.99	25	63	27	50		8	12	15	12	50	33	0	1	4
57	24.02.99	25.08.99	21	63	57	32	2	12	34	28	29	54	62	0	4	6
57	24.02.99	02.12.99	13	54	57	40	0	13	28	28	17	42	71	1	8	9
57	24.02.99	02.03.00	21	63	50	40	0	10	30	38	21	75	46	1	5	12
57	24.02.99	13.07.00	42	71	43	46	0	20	29	50	12	42	42	5	5	31
57		20.09.01	50	92	70	52		15	40	43	33	67	75			
58	11.03.99	07.06.99	25	71	43	38	2	14	25	29	12	38	42	4	1	5
58	11.03.99	04.10.99	71	96	57	42	0	18	27	28	38	33	58	0	0	12
58	11.03.99	07.02.00	42	83	70	44	4	11	20	29	29	25	29	1	0	14
58		22.05.00	58	96	40	56	0	15	20	31	8	21	21	0	3	22
58	11.03.99	22.05.00	58	96	40	56	0	15	20	31	8	21	21	0	2	22
58		30.07.01	56	80	60	54	4	10	15	26	17	38	42	0	1	9
59	18.03.99	24.06.99	50	96	50	50	4	8	36	34	12	50	67	5	17	36
59		12.10.99	25	63	62	42	0	11	34	38	21	71	75	0	12	19
59		17.02.00	33	79	50	40	0	15	38	49	21	75	54	0	12	22
59		26.05.00	46	92	57	48	0	9	34	53	25	75	79	3	21	32
60	20.04.99	29.07.99	29	83	46	34	0	28	41	55	21	46	62	0	29	48
60		17.01.00	33	88	57	51	0	20	27	50	46	67	79	2	21	42
60		01.05.00	38	100	57	54	0	30	51	65	46	67	79	0	18	48
60		04.06.01	54	96	70	58		20	35	60	46	79	83	6	44	54
61	27.04.99	07.07.99	54	88	57	64	0	26	46	55	29	71	54	1	31	72
61	27.04.99	06.12.99	63	83	63	68	0	34	40	59	38	67	88	5	44	83
61	27.04.99	20.06.00	63	92	67	62	2	26	41	69	46	62	67	9	48	73
62	14.05.99	19.08.99	17	75	37	36	0	10	22	34	21	42	46	0	24	33
62		22.11.99	38	75	38	40	0	15	39	40	29	67	54	2	16	23
62		02.03.00	13	79	53	35	0	10	34	38	25	46	62	0	15	31
62		09.10.00	29	79	20	24		12	52	48	21	54	79			
63	11.06.99	09.09.99	17	88	53	44	0	20	56	48	25	75	54	0	37	54
63		09.12.99	67	96	67	60	0	24	47	63	42	71	83	0	32	62
63		18.02.00	83	100	67	72	2	29	45	69	38	75	96	3	39	75
63		25.05.00	67	92	57	60	0	19	31	53	46	67	92	0	56	63
63		29.05.01	63	96	67	71		29	35	49	42	75	71	0	50	73
64	17.06.99	13.08.99	13	46	50	34	0	15	32	46	12	71	71	0	20	30
64		17.11.99	50	83	37	38	0	8	48	47	8	38	60	0	21	21
64		13.08.99	13	46	50	34	0	15	32	46	12	71	71	0	20	30
64		26.06.00	17	58	45	33	0	9	39	58	17	50	58	1	23	31
65	16.07.99	27.10.99	8	50	41	0	0	8	32	38	12	46	58	0	17	17
65		24.01.00	29	75	50	42	0	10	37	48	8	50	54	3	9	27
65		16.05.00	29	67	53	42	0	8	29	55	8	79	58	1	18	18
65		11.09.00	4	63		36		5	38	38	12		79			
65		11.12.00	25	54	47			8	37	49	17	58	71	0	14	16
66	26.08.99	30.09.99	17	58	30	24		5	25	23	12	67	62	0	22	15

abi mult otto alle nov01.html 30.03.2006 20:06 Uhr

66	26.08.99	09.02.00	8	54	30	36	0	4	31	36	21	33	58	1	25	20	
66		05.06.00	25	63	57	34	0	13	33	38	8	54	71	2	43	26	
66	26.08.99	16.11.00	50	75	73	68	0	28	34	44	25	67	79	3	27	47	
67	15.09.99	15.11.99	42	71	63	35	0	14	32	35	29	50	71	1	36	59	
67	15.09.99	24.04.00	29	83	57	40	0	11	54	64	21	62	75	5	38	50	
67		13.09.00	33	79	63	60		30		58	19		42				
68	22.10.99	14.12.99	17	38	43	19	0	0	0	0	0	0	0	0	0	0	
68		21.03.00	4	38	53	28	0	0	0	0	0	0	0	0	0	0	
68	22.10.99	28.09.00	13	50	43	36							21				
70	14.12.99	23.02.00	8	33	36	41	0	3	35	39	8	83	75	5	25	37	
70		10.07.00	21	67	41	22	0	16	41	56	17	88	88	5	18	23	
70		01.02.01	25	67	50	25		9		49	8	0	75				
70		31.05.01	17	75	40	36		7	37	43	17	75	67	5	24	34	
71	21.12.99	16.02.00	29	75	63	28	0	15	29	32	8	38	42	1	0	9	
71	21.12.99	30.05.00	21	71	27	50	2	22	25	48	21	42	54	2	2	15	
71	21.12.99	28.08.00	33	33	71	80	48	0	23	26	34	12	33	46	0	0	1
71		15.03.01	46	58	73	56		21	34	51	33	38	58	0	0	10	
74	08.02.00	13.06.00	17	54	43	38	0	9	7	22	21	33	38	0	11	17	
74	08.02.00	20.09.00	17	58	47	36		12	24	34	17	38	38	1	18	22	
74		11.01.01	8	29	43	32		12	22	29	25	38	42				
74		09.05.01	38	79	47	36		12	19	37	12	46	67	0	20	29	
75	03.05.00	13.07.00	13	79	47	26	2	14	27	30	8	54	71	0	36	50	
75		17.10.00	67	96	60	38	4	12	34	40	38	50	79	3	52	54	
75		16.01.01	46	88	53	52		9		49	33	50	83	3	52	54	
75		06.08.01	50	92	43	56		24			25						
76	09.05.00	28.08.00	25	54	47	35	0	19	30	50	17	67	67	0	19	48	
76		23.02.01	38	75	60	48		6		42	25		54				
76		01.06.01	38	88	70	54		8	43	43	33	75	92	0		27	
77	25.05.00	26.07.00	54	79	63	50	0	20	23	38	12	42	50	1	34	58	
77	25.05.00	26.10.00	80	100	63	86	2	34	38	66	12	79	75	10	21	78	
77		05.03.01	79	92	60	70		53	45	64	38	75	67	19	26	72	
77		04.06.01	79	96	80	80		44	35	66	41	75	83	19	37	87	
79	16.08.00	23.10.00	13	63	50	32		6	30	27	8	29	42	0	12	14	
79		09.08.01	21	88	60	37		12		41	0	50	46	0	10	31	
80	03.10.00	15.11.00	46	83	67	60											
81		06.03.01	13	58	57	28											
84		13.03.01	25	67	53	46		3	29	41	17	58	75				
84		19.06.01	42	83	60	42		14	34	48	8	75	83				
84		02.10.01	46	79	63	52		16	31	49	17	50	79	0	43	56	
85		20.03.01	33	83	67	44					8	58	71				
85		14.06.01	42	83	73	52		8	17	38	25	62	75				
86		24.04.01			70	40		13	30	48							
86		24.07.01	50	96	70	62		26	32	56	21	88	100				
86		24.10.01	54	96	77	56		25	40	55	29	79	83	3	33	69	
87		17.05.01	33	75	50	38		12	19	20	8	46	50	0	8	25	
87		07.08.01	79	100	50	68		11		12				3	11	42	
87		23.10.01	75	88	50	70	0	6	40	47	17	79	58	1	15	59	
88		18.07.01	25	71	43	26		11	29	50	21	54	50				
89		31.10.01	50	75	33	48		10	29	39	25	58	79	0	54	70	
92		19.09.01	54	92	63	58		21		51	17	54	67				

93	12.09.01	33	88	63	36		12	48	53	12	50	79			
94	16.10.01	4	50	47	42		2	18	33	4	46	75			
95	04.10.01	20	75	37	40				31			25			16

Herstellung und Verlag:
Books on Demand GmbH, Norderstedt
ISBN 978-3-8423-0034-7